# CHANGING
# HEALTH
# CARE

# CHANGING
# HEALTH
# CARE

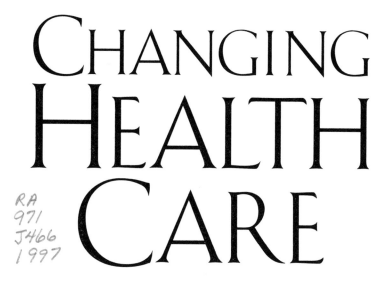

*Creating Tomorrow's
Winning Health
Enterprise Today*

ANDERSEN
CONSULTING

Ken Jennings, Ph.D.     Kurt Miller     Sharyn Materna

FOREWORD BY
Karen Ignagni
*President and CEO of the
American Association of Health Plans (AAHP)*

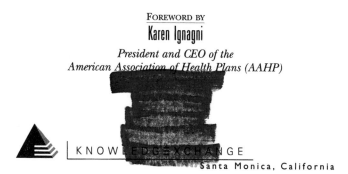

KNOWLEDGEXCHANGE

Santa Monica, California

**Knowledge Exchange, LLC**
**1299 Ocean Avenue**
**Santa Monica, California 90401**
TEL: **310.394.5995**
FAX: **310.394.7637**
E-MAIL: **kex@kex.com**
WEB: **http://www.kex.com**

Jacket design by Lee Fukui
Text design by Pirog Design

1 2 3 4 5 6 7 8 9-VA-99 98 97 96
First printing January 1997
ISBN: 1-888232-18-8

Knowledge Exchange books are available at special discounts for bulk purchases by corporations, institutions, and other organizations. For more information, please contact
Knowledge Exchange, LLC, at (310) 394-5995 (voice line) or kex@kex.com (e-mail).

# CONTENTS

# LIST OF FIGURES

# ACKNOWLEDGMENTS

*Changing Health Care* was truly a collaborative effort in that the named authors represent only a small part of the team involved in producing this book. Many of our friends and colleagues from within and outside of Andersen Consulting also made important contributions by acting as sounding boards and sharing their ideas, offering their knowledge as industry experts, critiquing various drafts, and assisting in personal interviews. Others worked diligently on the production and support of the book.

First and foremost, we want to thank the clients of Andersen Consulting who contributed their time and energy to this effort and who shared with us their successes and failures and the lessons learned from their own transformational change initiatives. In addition to providing the substance for this book, they have enriched our own perspectives by sharing these experiences with us.

Individuals who deserve special recognition for their efforts include Kedrick Adkins, Jim Anderson, Christi Blish, Ann Blocker, David Blume, Dr. Deleys Brandman, Tim Breaux, Jim Brennan, Willie Cheng, Cecilia Chua, Scott Cleary, Chris Dinnin, Dr. Michael Eliastam, Robert Friesen, Matthew Fust, Ed Giniat, Tony Hancy, Chuck Henderson, Jim Hudak, Julie Husband, T. Hardy Jackson, Stacey Jones, Wendy Kingsbury, Bob Lauer, Jenny Lehman, Ray Lenhardt, Janet Lorenz, Irene McFadden, Mike Manley, Rich Monroe, Terry Neill, Catherine Pettersson, Tom Prchal, Mike Rainey, David Rey, Bart Riley, Linda Ronan, Steve Rushing, Doug Ryckman, Jay Saddler, Marya Sakowicz Witt, Carl Schartner, Ash Shehata, Scott Soifer, Cindy Strazis, Ned Troup, Ann Van der Hijde, Shari Wenker, and Brian Younger. We are particularly grateful to David Osborn for his contribution to the Enablement chapter.

Special thanks go to Susan Vanderpool, who put in many long hours and a lot of energy assisting the authors in researching, coordinating information, interviewing, scheduling, creating presentations, and whatever else it took to bring this project to a successful conclusion.

In addition, special gratitude goes to Andersen Consulting's research and support team: Donna Carpenter, Erik Hansen, Bill Birchard, G. Patton Wright, Christina Braun, Morris Coyle, Elyse Friedman, Martha Lawler, Laura Pease, and Michelle Owen. We are also very grateful to Helen Rees, our energetic literary agent.

Finally, a special salute goes to the reviewers who offered excellent feedback: Kedrick Adkins, Jim Anderson, Paige Heavey, Jim Hudak, Phyllis Kennedy, Paul London, David Rey, and Carl Schartner.

# FOREWORD

## PUTTING PATIENTS FIRST: WHY HEALTH PLANS AND CONSUMERS ARE NATURAL PARTNERS

### Karen Ignagni

The revolution in health care today, a revolution of attitudes and expectations as much as of the organization and delivery of care, is as inevitable at the end of this century as the industrial revolution was at the beginning. And this revolution, like that one, has its opponents, who would much prefer to keep things as they were. But reversing a genuine revolution is as unlikely today as it was then.

Anyone who doubts that a revolution is taking place in health care should spend some time exploring the World Wide Web. Five years ago, that very idea would have been meaningless for most people—and for many it still is. The fact is, however, that there are millions of Americans who, when they need health care information, are likely to begin searching in cyberspace.

A remarkable array of online resources awaits them there. Browsing the Internet recently, the *New York Times* found 1,633 Web sites on medicine, 983 on diseases and conditions, 389 on pharmaceuticals, 346 on mental health, 194 on alternative medicine—and many, many more.

### *What do these numbers tell us?*

First, note that the numbers themselves were changing even as the *Times* was reporting them. New online sites are constantly appearing. Health plans, information services, medical-software firms, and others are creating a steadily growing cornucopia of new ventures, all of them designed to address consumers' seemingly insatiable demand for specific health information. And consumers themselves are organizing on-line services such as support groups for those with particular illnesses and ad hoc advisories about which health plans have the best reputations in a particular community.

It's clear that the exponential expansion of online health care information is an indicator of a sea change that is taking place in what once seemed to be an immutable relationship between health care professionals and their patients.

The old model was straightforward. The patient's role was to seek help when something went wrong. Doctors and hospitals provided the answers—and, after the advent of health insurance, sent their bills to a third party, which paid them, no questions asked.

That model can still be found, but it is diminishing by the day. The transformation of health care is far advanced. Purchasers of health care had a major role in triggering the revolution when they began questioning the escalating costs of coverage and care, but today individual consumers have the most to gain and are playing an increasingly important role. Although generalizations about a nation of more than 250 million individuals are always risky, it's clear that very large numbers of us are choosing to become more active partners in maintaining our health and managing illness.

For many Americans, the days are gone of passively assuming that someone else always has the answers. When health care questions arise today, a consumer armed with a computer and a modem has access to information as wide-ranging as that of a medical school library, as current as this week's medical journals, and as interactive as a conversation among friends. As a result, opportunities abound for more active partnerships between caregivers and patients.

On both sides of the patient-caregiver alliance, this is a revolution being driven by information. One hesitates to speak of "the information age," because that phrase and others like it are so overworked. But in the case of health care, it's really no exaggeration to say that we are just now entering the age of shared information, and the full implications of that shift are only just now beginning to be widely appreciated.

For health plans, the timing could hardly be more fortuitous. Today's integrated health care networks have always relied on information, of course, but they have only recently arrived at the point of being able to make much of it meaningful for purchasers and patients. Today, performance measures that were once considered to be beyond the reach of meaningful data analysis—or, at the very least, proprietary— are being converted into increasingly consumer-friendly report cards that can be used to compare everything from immunization rates to surgical outcomes. And today's report cards are just a start compared with what will soon become feasible as health plans become ever more proficient at capturing, interpreting, and sharing relevant data about prevention, acute and chronic care practices, and outcomes. Tomorrow's consumers will have, at their electronically enhanced fingertips, more information about more aspects of health care than anyone could have imagined even a few years ago.

But we should not lose sight of the fact that information, in and of itself, is like the famous tree that falls in the forest. What kind of sound it makes depends on who hears it. The impact of information depends on who is using it and for what purpose.

This fact has special relevance for health plans because of the related fact that so many of our patients are new to the kind of health care we practice. We can't afford the luxury of assuming they understand how we work. On the contrary, all the evidence suggests that significant numbers of health plan participants are unfamiliar with the advantages of health care networks—and thus especially susceptible to misinformation.

And that makes perfect sense when you consider how swiftly our world has changed. Twenty-five years ago, "health maintenance organization" was a newly coined phrase, and not one American in ten would likely have been able to say what the acronym "HMO" stood for. Ten years ago, HMO membership stood at 25.7 million, but that was still only one American out of every nine, and HMO enrollment was highly concentrated in a few states. Today, the more than 1,000 HMOs, PPOs, and similar plans that make up the membership of the American Association of Health Plans provide health care to more than 100 million Americans, and the total number of people receiving care through such plans reached an estimated 149 million in 1995—which represented an increase of 13 percent over the previous year's figure.

These numbers offer persuasive proof that HMOs and PPOs have long since moved from the margins of health care to the mainstream. But the very rapid growth in the number of Americans receiving care through HMOs and PPOs means that, at any given moment, a significant percentage of patients are new to our system of health care. As recent arrivals, they may feel a bit disoriented. They do not necessarily know their way around. They may even be anxious about how they will be cared for.

Health plans may be forgiven for feeling confident that their way of delivering care is the best way, but humility has its advantages. If we think of every new member as someone to be won over, we are likely to do a much better job of reaching out to them.

And the inescapable fact is that we must compete for their loyalty. That doesn't end when they sign up. It is an ongoing, daily process, and it involves more than one kind of competition.

There is, of course, intense—and healthy—competition within the industry. But there is also competition for the loyalty of consumers from those who oppose our entire philosophy of care.

Advocates of the old-style fee-for-service system are unlikely to be able to turn back the clock entirely, because there is just too much evidence that the nation cannot afford a system of health care that is essentially unaccountable with respect to quality as well as cost. But they can still do a great deal of damage, selectively using atypical horror stories to make generalized indictments of our approach to care. And every one-sided account of denial of care becomes grist for the mills of those who would like to limit health care networks by one means or another, whether by prohibiting capitation or requiring plans to contract with any willing provider.

The solution to this problem is the same whether communicating with consumers or with the media. Health plans should operate on the assumption that every encounter has the potential to turn out well or poorly, and that the outcome cannot be taken for granted. A corollary assumption is that no encounter should be regarded as trivial or routine.

This point can be illustrated by drawing on what we know from countless consumer satisfaction surveys. As a rule, the longer a patient remains with a health plan, the higher the level of satisfaction. The importance of this finding would be hard to exaggerate. It confirms what we intuitively know: that it is the new member who is most likely to be anxious and unfamiliar with the system—and, therefore, most vulnerable to misinformation.

Consider just a few of the questions that new members ask: What is a primary care physician? How do I pick one? What do you mean, my urologist can't be my primary care physician? I know it was a false alarm, but why is my trip to the emergency room not being paid? What's all this I hear about gag rules? Is it true my doctor can't talk to me about the treatment I need because you don't cover it? Is it true what I hear about my doctors making more money by not taking care of me? Is that what capitation means?

These questions have several things in common. They all reflect varying degrees of unfamiliarity with how health plans really work. They all reflect skepticism about whether health plans are more focused on the bottom line than on patient care and quality outcomes. They all reflect anxiety, which in any case is never far removed when the topic is health care. And they are all ticking time bombs. The health plan that ignores questions like these or takes them for granted is not only doing a disservice to its members, it is also shortening its own life expectancy and making life unnecessarily difficult for every other health plan.

The answer—remembering what our consumer satisfaction surveys tell us about the satisfaction curve rising with the duration of membership—is to treat the new member like a prospective member or anyone else who may have had no contact whatsoever with a health plan. The answer, in short, is that health care is an ongoing campaign. And the core concept in that campaign, just as in our philosophy of care, must be to always put the patient first.

Recognizing this, AAHP and its member plans recently drafted and ratified a statement that summarizes, in plain language, the principles that form our philosophy of care, and we are using this statement as the centerpiece of our platform in our ongoing campaign to strengthen the patient-plan relationship. Our philosophy of care focuses on quality, accountability, partnership, choice, prevention, and affordability—all the issues that are crucial to patients and that are hallmarks of our philosophy of care. After all, this is the philosophy we live by, the philosophy that has made our approach to health care so timely and successful, and this is information that we want patients to have—whether they read it in a health plan's literature or on a card in a waiting room, or reported in their local newspaper, or on an electronic bulletin board.

As should be clear by now, one of the explicit assumptions behind this campaign is that health care consumers are changing—that they are not the least reticent about seeking out information, that they are rightly skeptical of any attempt to withhold it or distort it, and that they will become natural allies and partners of health plans that meet their needs.

That being the case, the challenge for health plans—in a highly competitive marketplace—is clear. Plans that master the total information environment will have a decided advantage over those that do not. But what does a phrase like "total information environment" encompass?

To illustrate, consider these hypothetical points along the online information spectrum:

▼ My employer offers me a choice of three plans. I want to make a detailed comparison of benefits, right down to comparing coverage of specific drugs and specific pre-existing conditions. Two of the plans provide general but not very detailed brochures. I can't seem to find what I'm looking for. The third plan offers an interactive, constantly updated online service addressing dozens of Frequently Asked Questions (FAQs). In less than ten minutes I find what I'm looking for. Which plan am I likely to choose?

▼ I'm concerned about my diabetic sister. Although she's not covered by my plan, when I access my plan's Web site, I'm guided to all kinds of useful information. With a few keystrokes, I order an educational videotape and have it sent to her. A year later, she has joined my plan and reports that she's receiving wonderful health guidance. When the opportunity to switch plans arises, I think about this kind of service and decide to stay where I am.

▼ My mother, who has osteoporosis, is interested in switching from traditional Medicare coverage to a coordinated-care plan, but she's confused about what her out-of-pocket costs will be and whether she'll be able to arrange for physical therapy at home after hip surgery. My daughter, the family computer jockey, offers to do some online research. She learns about a plan that, in addition to arranging all at-home physical therapy needs, offers a free "home health audit" to help identify hazards that could cause a fall or other injury. "Mom," I say, "I think we've found the plan for you."

▼ We're moving to a new city, and we'll be traveling a lot. Online, we compare the doctors affiliated with our plan in our new location and verify their availability. We do the same with hospitals. And we run across an online news story about how our plan, despite being based in the Midwest, arranged complete care for a family—including special care on a flight home—after they suffered multiple injuries in a car crash while vacationing in Latin America. The story makes us feel very good about our choice of plans.

As it happens, all of these examples involve true-to-life interactions between consumers and plans that, to one degree or another, would have been problematic if not out of the question just a few years ago. All of them have a bearing on how consumers determine value in selecting and using health plans. And all of them are related to how imaginatively a plan manages the vast array of information resources at its command.

This is, of course, an evolutionary process. Beginning with the first rudimentary attempts to capture and assess patient-plan encounter data, health plans steadily expanded the horizons of internal information management. Then, working with major corporate purchasers of health care, they began developing better quality-measurement tools. Today, even as the evolution of data-based quality assessment continues, they are in a position to share this information with—and to make it meaningful for—individual consumers. And once again, for many reasons, the timing could not be more fortuitous.

From the standpoint of national policy, the overriding challenge in the years ahead is to continue transforming our health care delivery system so that it consistently delivers optimum value: superior quality and coverage at predictable, acceptable cost. Critics argue that health plans can manage costs only by limiting access to care. Aside from ignoring all the contrary evidence, that view either overlooks or underrates the myriad opportunities to improve care and control costs by building real partnerships—shared-information partnerships—between health plans and consumers.

The benefits of such partnerships should be readily apparent. The young mother-to-be who connects to a comprehensive prenatal care network becomes a better-informed patient, improving the odds of a normal, uncomplicated delivery. Clinically, that means a better outcome. Societally, it means lower cost. And it can happen because of a health plan's aggressive commitment to outreach—which, in turn, is information-driven.

Outreach doesn't just happen. It has to take place within and as part of a plan's total operational commitment to continual quality improvement. Management must constantly ask (and strive to answer) such tough questions as the following.

Why aren't we experiencing more normal deliveries? How do we reach more mothers? Is it easy for them to reach us?

How long does it take them to get through when they call us? Does the person who takes their call answer their questions? How long does it take to make an appointment with a physician? How long is the typical waiting-room wait? Are they getting first-class care? Did someone follow up after the visit? Do they regularly receive helpful literature from us? Can they find answers 24 hours a day? Online? Does everything we do make them feel welcome, or do we come across as just another big, impersonal, indifferent organization?

All of these questions are thoroughly interconnected; the answers to all of them will turn on how well or poorly a health plan is handling and integrating its information-gathering, information-management, and information-dissemination functions. And in health care, as in other fields, one can safely assume that not all organizations have mastered the art and science of handling the entire information infrastructure with state-of-the-art expertise.

The stakes are, of course, enormous. The transformation of health care is an ongoing process in which the momentum of change is, if anything, accelerating. As more and more Americans of all ages make the shift from old-style fee-for-service coverage to coordinated-care plans, more and more consumers will be unwilling to settle for anything less than a genuine working partnership with the health plan they choose.

Health care professionals can be forgiven for wondering whether they are entirely prepared for this kind of partnership. To a degree, at least, they may feel that they are in uncharted territory—and they are right. In that situation, it would help to have a reliable guide. Now they do.

*Changing Health Care* could not be more timely. Gathered here, in one well-conceived and wide-ranging volume, are many insights on the conceptual challenges facing health care management professionals today, accompanied by scores of examples of how leading health plans are transforming themselves to ensure that they will still be leading the way tomorrow.

As the authors emphasize, this transformation process can involve a high degree of uncertainty even under the best of circumstances. In a field as complex as health care—a sector of the economy that is, itself, larger than the economies of most nations—there is no foolproof way to guarantee strategic competitiveness. But the odds can surely be greatly improved if an organization can develop the capacity to examine its internal strengths and weaknesses at the same time that it studies and responds to the marketplace. The great strength of *Changing Health Care* is that it can help health plans to do both. Readers will not necessarily agree with every idea they encounter here, but they will find this a singularly challenging and thought-provoking book.

*Changing Health Care* demonstrates decisively that the successful health care organization of the future will be, above all, nimble. As the authors warn, a needlessly multilayered bureaucracy will not serve as a model, and the oldest of maxims—"we've always done it this way"—will not suffice as a corporate motto. Instead, innovative health plans and health care professionals will work together to create, and sustain, partnerships with consumers that are firmly based on mutual respect and understanding.

Flexibility is crucial for many reasons, but most of all because consumers want different things at different times. A young, healthy family with few health care issues may want primarily ease of access to reliable information and preventive-care appointments. Someone who has just been given an alarming diagnosis, on the other hand, needs more than information; he or she needs to feel connected to a network of caring people who are capable of listening, responding, and guiding the patient to and through the appropriate treatment options. And a patient facing a long or chronic illness needs the peace of mind that comes with knowing that all necessary services will be provided—at the right time, in the right setting, and without bureaucratic hassles—by a health plan that will be there tomorrow, not just today.

The health care organization that meets only some of these needs may survive, but it will not be the health plan of choice for informed consumers. They will gravitate instead to a health plan that meets them more than half way: a plan that anticipates their needs and earns their continuing allegiance.

It is in addressing that side of the health care equation— the consumer demand side—that *Changing Health Care* performs a real public service. Much attention has been paid, by the media and others, to changes on the supply side: to the replacement of fee-for-service by coordinated care and to the implications of delivering health care through regional and national networks. Too little attention has been paid to how health care is being and will be changed on the demand side by the emergence of consumers who are comfortable with information technologies, who are aware of the importance of maintaining their health as well as managing their illnesses, and who—in their search for the optimum balance of coverage, quality, and cost—won't be reluctant to comparison-shop.

That is a healthy change, and this book is a healthy addition to the literature of network-based, consumer-driven health care. It confirms what we at AAHP deeply believe: that consumers and health plans committed to putting patients first are natural partners.

*Karen Ignagni is President and CEO of the American Association of Health Plans (AAHP), the national association of health maintenance and preferred provider organizations. Based in Washington, D.C., AAHP can be reached at http://www.aahp.org on the World Wide Web.*

# INTRODUCTION

A personal adventure in health care for an overconfident management consultant began with a challenging white water rafting trip. The class four and five rapids on the New River in West Virginia caused his L5-S1 lumbar disk to rupture badly. Neurosurgery was performed at a busy university hospital, a client of his at that time. Despite the pain and severity of the injury, the patient/management consultant believed the surgery was a chance to assess the benefits of transforming traditional practices in health care. He even took notes every step of the way, from the physician's office to surgical preparation, to postoperative recovery.

That consultant, as you have probably guessed, was one of us (Ken Jennings). Just two months earlier, we helped physicians and the university hospital reengineer the lumbar laminectomy process. The experience shows—rather vividly— that in our years of consulting we have managed to see health care from a wide variety of viewpoints, even as patients on operating tables. It is the breadth of these viewpoints, along with the collective experience of our numerous colleagues at Andersen Consulting, that has yielded many of the insights you are about to read.

We have not limited our research to picking the brains of the organizations and people we already know well. We have taken care to draw on the wisdom of the best and brightest minds from throughout the health care industry. Most notably, we have benefited from a gold mine of leadership provided by scores of one-on-one interviews conducted with people at all organizational levels of health care organizations, from an elite roster of chief executives to the dedicated ranks of clerks and care givers on the front lines.

Following are the stories of these people who are helping to invent the future of health care. They will engage and inspire you with their vision, their commitment, their innovations. But more important, they will help us reveal for you our blueprint for transforming your organization into a winning health care enterprise.

The argument we present here is straightforward and practical. It has three conceptually distinct parts: creating winning strategies, building key competencies, and managing the journey of change. The three parts interconnect like a chain, one link locked inextricably with the next, each essential for organizational excellence. Together, the three links will enable health care organizations to prosper as they try to meet the challenges of the years ahead.

None of the three links in this chain of excellence will, alone, enable organizations to turn themselves into the winning health care enterprises of the future. For example, an organization can establish breakthrough strategies, but competitors can duplicate or counter those strategies. An organization can develop exceptional competencies, but competitors can replicate or buy those competencies. An organization can even develop the capability for massive change, but competitors can develop the same change management skills. The key to becoming a winning health care enterprise of the future is to create an unbroken connection among all three: Successful enterprises will win by crafting innovative strategies, enabling them with world-class competencies, and executing both with outstanding skills in change management.

Although in our research we rarely found organizations that had forged a strong three-part chain of excellence, many will have to learn how to do so, because the question of whether a revolution will force change in health care is moot: The revolution is already here, driven by an extraordinary array of forces. Foremost is the requirement for health care organizations to deliver far more value to health care consumers.

The health care consumer, to borrow an old cliché, is becoming king. Organizations are now facing a new consumer of health care—new because of an increased access to clinical and medical knowledge through the Internet and information technology, new because of an invigorated attitude about the need to monitor one's own health status, engage in wellness programs, and seek alternative medicines and treatments. These new consumers of health—whether individuals, employers, or other health care organizations—now wield tremendous power, directing not only what changes occur in this revolution but also how organizations will operate in the coming decades. The ability to identify these consumers and anticipate their needs is a vital capability for the winning health organization.

## Part I: *Driving Forces and Winning Strategies*

Because the first step in transforming your organization into a winning enterprise is setting strategy, we have dedicated the first section of our book to outlining five strategies (Figure 1) for positioning your enterprise as a leader in the industry.

▼ Keep ahead of consumers: Create a continuous stream of innovations in products and services that result in unmatched value.

▼ Cut to the moment of value: Eliminate all non-value-adding processes, middlemen, and barriers to effective health care.

▼ Give your best and virtualize the rest: Partner with other organizations to offer customers the highest-quality continuum-of-care services.

***Figure 1*** Winning Strategies

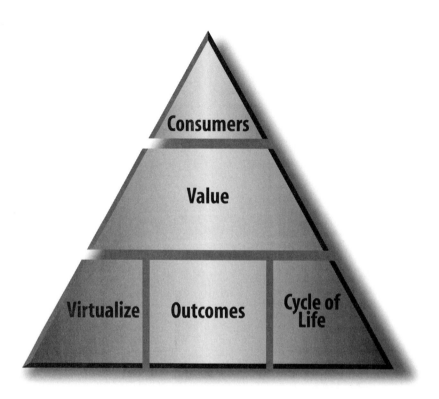

▼ Mine the riches of outcomes: Capture and analyze data for any process, treatment, service, or product that brings true value to customers.

▼ Mind the cycle of life: Design and market products and services that prevent illness, enhance health, and ease the debilitating effects of illness and disease.

In our studies of health care organizations throughout the United States and the world, we found that winners are those who use these five strategies (or a version of them) to create unprecedented excellence in providing value for customers.

## Part II: *Key Competencies*

In the second part of our book, we discuss four key competencies (Figure 2) that support the strategies for developing a competitive advantage. These competencies combine the requisite elements of technology, processes, and human capital to execute them.

▼ ***Liberating the health care consumer:*** Health care organizations must establish friendly, productive, and trusting relationships with their plan members and patients. They must

***Figure 2*** WINNING COMPETENCIES

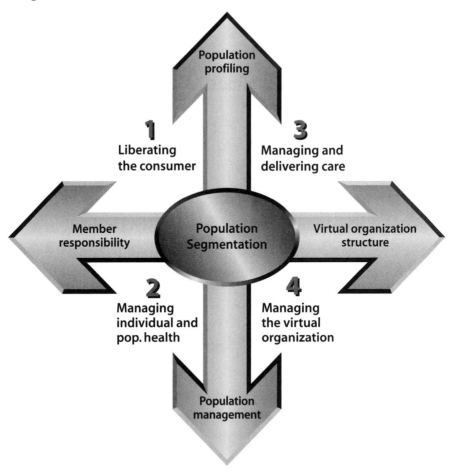

empower individual consumers with the information and incentives they need to enhance their own health status and make smart access and utilization choices.

▼ *Managing individual and population health:* It is no longer sufficient to excel at curing maladies and insuring against catastrophic loss. Winning health enterprises must focus on customized wellness programs, prevention, and proactive management of health risks and chronic conditions.

▼ *Managing and delivering care:* This competency can be characterized as a combination of four essential elements: providing the right service in the right setting by the right person using the right processes. It is enabled through the use of protocols, teams, and virtualized service delivery and includes triage services, care management and delivery, appointment scheduling, referral management, and other administrative "touch" processes to better serve consumers.

▼ *Aligning the services and resources of the virtual organization:* Winning health enterprises must develop the ability to make the virtual organization a reality. Few health care enterprises are able to provide all the services, products, treatments, care paths, and wellness centers that their customers want or need. Instead, they must build alliances and partnerships based on mutually beneficial approaches, shared values, shared information, aligned incentives, and revised governance models.

## Part III:  *Change Management*

We devote the third section of our book to change management and execution, perhaps the most critical of the competencies of the successful health care organization. In our studies of various organizations—managed care firms, pharmaceutical companies, integrated delivery systems, physician management organizations, and the like—we discovered impressive innovations in strategies and excellence in building competencies. We also found organizations that had exceptional success in executing programs and services. But we found the real winners to be those enterprises that supported their strategies with real competencies and executed the changes needed to create those competencies.

The alignment of all three—strategies, competencies, and execution—cannot be had cheaply. This alignment is a function of relentless effort. In schematic form, the change man-

***Figure 3*** THE CHANGE MANAGEMENT FRAMEWORK

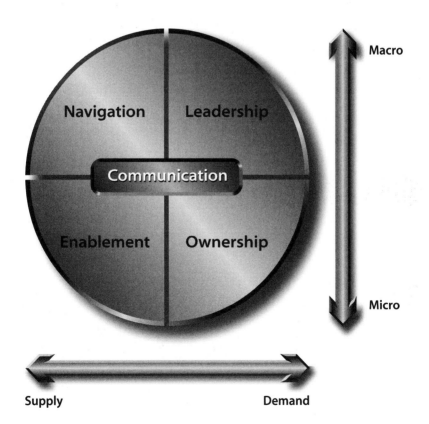

agement methodology, the third link in the chain of excellence, comprises four parts (Figure 3).

*Leadership* requires that managers inspire and guide the change. They must nurture a relentless commitment to the change and possess the resolve to follow it through to its final destination.

*Ownership* demands that managers sell the change and create demand that will insure buy-in. When people inside the organization understand why change is necessary and how they will benefit, their initial resistance will abate. Managers must implement innovative programs that inform and involve employees, members, and others who demand the organization's products and services.

*Enablement* calls on managers to deliver new systems, skills, and business processes that allow people to work more efficiently and effectively. This includes developing or updating training programs, strategies to support performance, job definitions, human-resource policies, and organizational structures. The goal is to equip everyone in the organization to embrace the new regime.

*Navigation* requires that managers take a holistic approach to coordinating all components of the change program. The goal is to develop a master plan for changing the organization, monitoring success, and adjusting the scope, pace, and risk as change initiatives progress.

We designed *Changing Health Care* to be a guidebook to the future, detailing the comprehensive and coordinated steps needed for the transformation of the health care enterprise and, ultimately, of the health care industry itself. In writing this book, we found real heroes in the health care industry, people who have committed themselves to the creation of winning enterprises. Their best practices serve as models for us all. We also found entire organizations that meet challenges head on, welcoming change as an opportunity to reinvent themselves. These organizations and those that join them in bravely stepping forward will become tomorrow's leaders, transforming themselves and the industry by making—and delivering on—bold promises.

Other organizations will be swept away, forced to accept subordinate roles in the newly integrated system or to survive as shadows of their former selves. Some institutions we know today will disappear altogether. Having grown complacent and overconfident, they will fail to notice that shifts in technology, customer base, and other forces for change are converging as megatrends that demand dramatic and quick responses. Slow to awaken and even slower to change, they will insist on keeping their systems' components independent rather than incorporating them into larger systems.

Few organizations today can survive and prosper in the midst of the health care revolution without undergoing transformation, without creating entire new businesses, without inventing new processes, new management systems, and new ways of seeing the future. In *Changing Health Care,* we demonstrate how you can lead your health care organization through that transformation, profiting both from the journey itself and from the destination. The kinds of transformation described in this book are made possible by dedicated individuals who execute their jobs with brilliance. We hope their stories will help you feel you are among them and serve as an inspiration during your journey of change.

Ken Jennings

Kurt Miller

Sharyn Materna

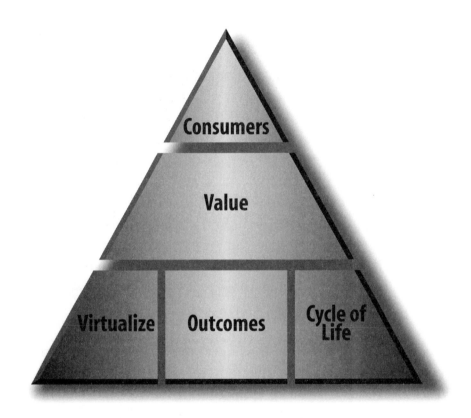

# PART I

## DRIVING FORCES AND WINNING STRATEGIES

# 1

## THE FORCES FOR CHANGE

A decade of fiery diatribe by increasingly aggressive health care payers and consumers has spurred a world of change in health care organizations. Stung by complaints over high costs, insurers have introduced products with prices so low they make heads turn. Blue Cross and Blue Shield of Oregon, for example, recently announced a new health care policy for the children of parents with low annual incomes: For only $29.50 a month, barely enough to cover its costs, BCBS/Oregon provides basic health care benefits for those children until they reach their eighteenth birthday. Most other insurers offer monthly coverage that costs up to 50 percent more. BCBS/Oregon has devised a strategy that sets the company apart from its competitors by providing unparalleled value for customers. That innovation simultaneously introduces a major risk and creates a major opportunity for the insurer. (Koco 1994)

Concerned about criticism of quality, managed care companies, such as United HealthCare based in Minnetonka, Minnesota, have built sophisticated systems to measure and continually improve the quality of care. In Milwaukee, United cut by 85 percent the number of asthmatic children rushed each year to the hospital. It accomplished that feat by first using computer-intensive data gathering to identify the troubling hospitalization pattern. It then created programs to encourage better management of medication and nebulizer use. (United HealthCare 1994)

Smarting from attacks on the mediocre levels of community health, hospitals such as Hackley Hospital in Muskegon, Michigan, have rushed to offer brand new outreach services. The 228-bed Hackley Hospital opened a community care center to give primary care to underserved local residents. In a county with a 1992 infant mortality rate of 14.4 percent, the hospital opened rehabilitation centers in two local fitness centers and has developed plans to establish wellness centers throughout the community. (Rauber 1994: 75, 76)

Governments, employers, and individual citizens worldwide continue to press the health care industry for satisfaction. A 1991 survey of attitudes in ten developed countries revealed that, with the exception of Canadians, less than 50 percent of people responding to a survey believed that their health care system "on the whole works pretty well and requires only minor changes to make it work better" (see Figure 4). The U.S. was dead last in the survey, and Canada's rating, while at the top of the heap, leaves plenty of room for improvement.

Although these studies illustrate chiefly consumers' judgments, they reflect what most of us associated with the health care industry know, only too well, to be true: Consumers today feel that they are not getting the value they deserve for the

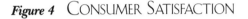
***Figure 4*** CONSUMER SATISFACTION

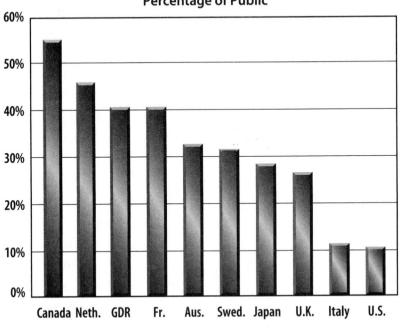

*Source: Blendon et al., 1990*

money they and their health care purchasers pay. Whereas
U.S. employers once paid much of the cost for health insurance, they now require their employees to supplement
monthly payments to insurers. Companies that used to pick
up all the costs of managed care health plans now demand a
$10–35 co-payment from their employees for each visit to a
physician. And where deductibles of $100 were once com-
mon, they now range as high as $1,000 or more. Consumers
pay more, wait longer, and demand more.

Payers, too, are feeling the crunch. For the past two
decades, U.S. health care spending has climbed five percentage points faster than the rate of inflation. Although in recent
years these increases have slowed, Americans spend double
the amount of money on health care that citizens of many

other developed countries spend. In 1950, health care spending constituted a mere 45.9 percent of educational spending. Today, it commandeers 14 percent of the gross domestic product, hundreds of billions of dollars. Translated into amounts we can better comprehend, roughly $2,000 of the cost of every new car produced in the United States is now attributable to the health care benefits that automobile manufacturers have to pay for their workers.

Of course, consumerism and the "big ugly health care buyer" are not the only pressures giving health care managers a headache. Also weighing on their minds are pressures from changing markets, new technology, profit hungry investors, shifting political winds, and new legal mandates. But as much as these pressures sometimes squeeze to the foreground, consumers are gaining control of the levers of power. They—as well as the plan sponsors who purchase health care coverage on their behalf and the new market entrants that clearly see the opening—are driving a fundamental revolution within the health care industry.

These pressures are part of a larger set of forces that are shaping health care worldwide as we move toward the new millennium. Winning health enterprises now embrace and leverage these forces to their advantage, while others continue to ignore them, often at their own peril. Driven by concerns over cost, quality, and service, these dramatic changes are occurring in health care systems throughout the developed world.

In a recently conducted study in countries throughout Europe, North America, and Asia, Andersen Consulting identified five key themes around which much of this industry-level transformation is occurring:

▼ *The new consumerism:* Traditional payers, such as governments and employers, are shifting more and more of the cost burden directly to consumers. At the same time, individuals are taking on increased responsibility and control of their own health care. Motivated by greater concern for their own health and a growing distrust of the traditional health care system, they are turning, in growing numbers, to alternative sources for advice and treatment. Armed with new technology, previously restricted access to medical information, and a much more health-savvy attitude, today's health care consumers are critical, aggressive, and knowledgeable, with every intention of prying open the stranglehold that certain insurance companies, HMOs, and providers have had on care.

▼ *Regional integrated delivery networks:* More and more health care organizations and governmental groups realize they cannot deliver the breadth and quality of services citizens and employers are demanding on their own. In the United States they are banding together in various ways—through mergers and acquisitions to create larger vertically structured enterprises or through partnerships and virtual unions powered by information technology—to provide integrated health care whenever and wherever it is needed. In countries with largely social health care systems, hospitals, physicians, and other providers, as well as insurers in some cases, are being privatized and grouped into systems such as Regional Health Corporations in Canada and Regional Health Authorities in New Zealand.

▼ *Cost management:* To control costs, many public and private sector payers are utilizing various forms of spending caps. In the United States, capitation, or a set fee per person, is allocated by or to the health care organization, or a set price is established for certain procedures or treatments. In countries with socialized medicine, global spending caps may determine when hospitals are closed or beds are taken out of service.

▼ *Competition to improve quality:* Health care organizations worldwide are increasingly utilizing various measures of quality as a basis for competition and allocation of funds. In the United States, for example, a number of health care organizations, such as Kaiser Permanente and United HealthCare, have issued quality "report cards," to provide information that consumers and other organizations can use to determine value.

▼ *The information infusion:* Information technology today is being used to reinvent care management and delivery processes in dramatic ways. For example, in the past the care giver, the patient, and the patient chart had to converge at a place and point in time for care to be delivered and received. These constraints of time, place, and form, however, are rapidly disappearing as technologies such as telemedicine, electronic medical records, telepresence, and the health care information superhighway enable care to be virtualized. Soon, health care will be available at any time, in any place.

These themes run throughout this book and provide the catalyzing energy for many of the stories, changes, and innovations you will read about. They are clearly evident in the United States and account, in large part, for the dynamic and sweeping changes occurring in various markets across the country. Figure 5 provides a framework for marking, measuring, and anticipating some of these changes. This figure also depicts the evolutionary path that many industries follow from nascence to maturity: Phase I, typically characterized by a limited set of fairly standard products, where price is the primary competitive weapon; Phase II, where market segmentation and keen insights into customer values enable organizations to craft highly targeted and focused offerings for specific

***Figure 5*** MARKET EVOLUTION PHASES

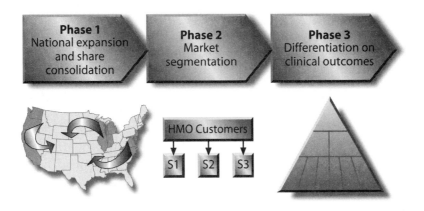

customer segments; and ultimately Phase III, where industry-wide quality standards are defined and measured, establishing an entirely new platform for competition.

Examples of all three phases exist in different markets throughout the United States. In many of these markets most health plans and providers are still focused largely on Phase I activities. The health care players in the Cleveland, Ohio, market, for example, provide a dramatic illustration. In an effort to increase market share and reduce costs, the care delivery system has experienced a massive transformation. In 1994, fourteen hospitals and four hospital systems were consolidated into three delivery networks. Consolidation among both providers and health plans has also occurred in the California and Minneapolis markets, and many other U.S. markets are undergoing similar changes.

Phase II activities revolve around market segmentation. During this phase competitive differentiation is often achieved by developing deeper insights into customers' needs and values, identifying specific market segments, and developing products and services targeted to each segment. Price is still a necessary element during this phase, but it alone is insufficient to ensure competitive advantage. It is simply an ante to stay in the game.

There are many examples of Phase II activities occurring throughout various markets. For our purposes, however, we will focus on the two types that appear to be most pervasive: first, those that offer expanded options in basic health plan products and benefits; second, those that offer differentiated, stand-alone products and services.

Among the earliest examples of health plan product segmentation, the point-of-service plans allow subscribers to receive services from out-of-network providers for a higher co-payment or deductible. Building on this type of product, several health plans are beginning to think more broadly about how to segment their customers in terms of overall product offerings. They are using techniques such as conjoint analysis to better understand how consumers make choices and balance trade-offs between factors such as price, choice, and service quality. Such analyses can assist them in developing marketing strategies and delivery networks specifically targeting each segment.

The second type of segmentation is taking shape with breathtaking speed across the country, although for many traditional industry players it still lies just off their competitive radar screens. Almost daily, new market entrants introduce new products and services targeted at various customer segments. Pharmaceutical companies, long beholden to the physician, now appeal directly to consumers: They offer disease management products through retail pharmacy outlets and mail order, while demand management vendors, targeting high-risk patients, drive Wall Street valuations rivaling those of a number of traditional health plans. In addition, software, media, entertainment, and cable companies are getting in on the act, mass customizing content and delivery channels for specific customer segments. To reach consumers frustrated with Western medicine's mechanistic and narrow view of health, acupuncturists, herbalists, and homeopaths are collecting billions in out-of-pocket, discretionary spending by consumers. In fact, while many traditional players are focused largely on Phase I competition, these new market entrants are taking more and more of the high-margin revenue dollars out of the market each year.

Early Phase III activity is also under way in a number of markets; however, universally accepted quality standards and measurement capabilities are still years away. As the ability to define and measure true clinical outcomes develops, health service organizations will look beyond price and service to build new value propositions based on formulas including price, service, and quality. In this phase, winning health enterprises will be identified by their ability to measure and quantify true clinical outcomes. They will define a new standard of competitive advantage, as customers, with access to new technology, become much more savvy about health care delivery and outcomes. Early, although somewhat primitive, efforts in this direction, using proxies such as immunization and complication rates, already abound. The Pennsylvania Health Care Cost Containment Council, for example, now publishes a consumer report that covers hospital effectiveness in fifty-nine categories, ranging from tonsillectomies to craniotomies. Recently it published a list of all hospitals and doctors performing coronary bypass surgery, the number of surgeries performed, the cost, and death rates. One hospital charged $103,000 for the surgery, whereas another charged only $28,000. The higher price guaranteed no better results; in fact, the hospital that charged the lower price had a slightly lower mortality rate. (Jimenez 1995: 6)

While consumers continue to apply pressure for more value, many groups inside the health industry are doing the same. Much as the J. D. Power reports have done for the automobile industry, those issued by the National Committee for Quality Assurance (NCQA), a health care accrediting group, will give consumers more of the empirical evidence they need to choose health providers. The NCQA's first report in 1995 compared 21 major health plans in 36 categories. (Winslow 1995: B6)

Similar types of groups have cropped up across the United States. A number of employers in New England have developed a template of quality measures for the region's HMOs. After only a brief time in operation, the group has convinced several employers to make purchasing decisions based on data it provides. Such revolutionary tactics in the name of liberating the consumer will continue to pressure health care managers to find innovative ways to provide better service and higher quality.

The not-so-subtle and often painful shift of power to a consumer-focused rather than an enterprise-focused system is aptly depicted by Dr. Tom Ferguson's inverted power pyramid, reproduced in Figure 6. "The whole structure of medicine," says Ferguson, "has been based on the assumption that physicians have the current information and patients do not. The bottom line is, the consumer will have virtually all the information the professionals have. This is comparable to the way communism fell. Once people start getting in good communication, you won't be able to play the game in the same way." (Ferguson 1995)

With this kind of leverage by both the consumer and the large payers, the key to winning in health care is the same one that other industries have already discovered: Turn consumer ambivalence or displeasure into consumer delight. To accom-

***Figure 6*** INVERTING THE POWER PYRAMID

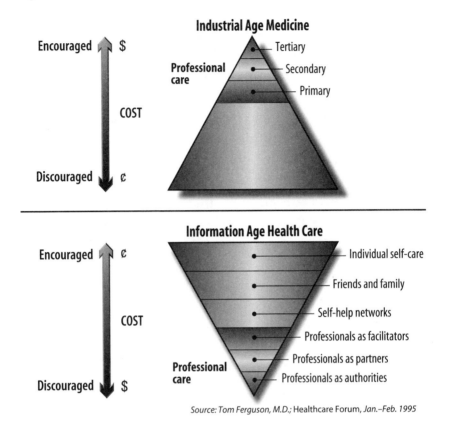

Source: Tom Ferguson, M.D.; Healthcare Forum, *Jan.–Feb. 1995*

plish this metamorphosis, today's health care enterprise must provide unprecedented value to consumers. But this value can occur only when organizations undertake changes to develop winning strategies supported by world-class competencies.

Understanding the management of change is a prerequisite for today's health care organizations to achieve competitive advantage. Many forces swirl—and occasionally collide—around them: New drugs and treatments make health care more efficient (and often more expensive), new threats to public health continue to emerge, and new corporate mergers and partnerships alter the list of players we have grown accustomed to seeing. Even in local hospitals, decision makers must think in global terms. Powerful technologies link players from every level and of every size to distant suppliers, patients, and providers.

When the Clinton administration's proposed health care reform plans were put on hold, the reaction throughout the industry was intense: Some resisted change altogether, adopting a "wait-and-see" attitude; some, panicking at the sight of minor wounds, chose to ignore the possibility of serious illnesses in their businesses; still others, taking radical steps, found themselves tripping over their own feet. But several organizations paused, took stock, and reacted quickly and rationally to sudden discontinuities in the marketplace:

▼ *Kaiser-Permanente:* This organization had an enviable franchise in the tough California market, but it decided to reinvent its approaches to service delivery. It is boldly turning its operations inside out and reengineering them from the members' point of view.

▼ *Physicians Health Service:* This midsize HMO in Connecticut decided to expand to New York State and the Big Apple by partnering with The Guardian, a traditional insurer. This highly unusual partnership took the market by storm and succeeded beyond even the planners' expectations.

▼ *Phycor and PacifiCare:* Phycor, a unique physician management company, and PacifiCare, a high-flying managed care organization, decided to grow by aggressively pursuing virtual organization strategies.

▼ *Baxter International:* Having established its reputation as a manufacturer of traditional medical products, Baxter International spun off a high-risk, $4.5 billion entity called Allegiance Healthcare Corporation to establish innovative partnerships with customers. Allegiance will comprise various businesses that can provide up to 80 percent of the products that hospitals and laboratories need, as well as cost-management services that can save health professionals millions of dollars annually.

▼ *Henry Ford Health System of Detroit, Michigan:* Gail Warden, the president and CEO of Henry Ford Health System, had seen his enterprise grow from a loose confederation of health care facilities into a large distribution network for a citywide HMO. Rejecting the temptation to abandon the city, Warden oversaw the extensive expansion of satellite facilities, which has transformed Henry Ford Health System into a thriving integrated patient care enterprise. "I have four objectives for this organization," Warden says. "They are the same this year as last year, and they will be the same next year: To be the low-cost provider with high-quality care; to achieve the greatest patient satisfaction; to continue to integrate the elements of the system; and to keep the focus on our customers." (Warden 1995)

▼ *Astra Merck, Inc.:* In 1993, two pharmaceutical giants— Merck and Company, Inc., and Astra AB of Sweden—created a new billion-dollar business from scratch. The new company facilitates the licensing of drugs developed by Astra and other pharmaceutical companies, then markets and sells the products in the United States. (Kiely 1993)

What do those organizations have in common? All of them are charting new courses as they fashion themselves into successful health care enterprises of the future. They accept huge risks by adopting major innovations in services, products, organizational structures, strategic partnerships, and alliances. Like many other organizations, they had, in the past, focused their attention on the provider, the procedure, or the health care organization's profits, while the members and the patients were lost in the shuffle. Today, however, those organizations are representative of the new leaders of an industry that is undergoing vast changes and upheavals.

In this section of the book, we describe the major forces driving the health care industry to change and to develop effective strategies for achieving success. We find that in fashioning their responses to those pressures, today's health care enterprises have shifted their focus to the patient and the customer. Indeed, the watchword in today's health care circles is customer value. And as so many industries have learned, value is the product of lower costs, higher quality, and, of course, better service.

Our interviews with health care professionals indicate that most people, inside and outside the industry, identify lower costs as the first element of customer value. No two ways about it, health care now and in the future is an expensive item, and there are horror stories galore illustrating needless expenditures and exorbitant prices. Consumers burn far more energy picking apart their bills than picking up on reasoned arguments from health care managers to justify costs. In spite of the unparalleled care many people now receive, many believe that a great portion of the exorbitant costs is avoidable if only the health care system could function economically. For example, critics point out that the United States spends a significant percentage of its health care bill on non-value-added administrative activities, such as moving mountains of paperwork between buyers, providers, and intermediaries. Other countries are able to accomplish these administrative tasks for a minimal percentage of their health care expenditures.

Critics also slam the industry for inappropriate care, particularly unnecessary medical tests and procedures. Care givers order duplicate tests or tests that are inappropriate to the patient's condition. Although there is much debate about what is necessary, a *Wall Street Journal* report estimated that $5–7 billion could be saved by routing patients to primary care physicians rather than treating them in hospital emergency rooms. (Winslow 1996) In addition, poorly informed patients sometimes request tests they do not need, despite their care givers' advice, and some health care professionals order tests that they believe to be unnecessary for medical reasons but necessary to avoid malpractice suits. All told, these tests and procedures can run up the U.S. health care tab by several billion dollars annually.

While conscious of the high costs, today's consumers still demand what from their point of view constitutes the highest-quality health care. And many consider it their right. To protect it, they are banding together in buyers' groups. More than 900,000 employees covered under the California Public Employees' Retirement System (CalPERS) benefited from the group's decision to identify and reward the health plans that best meet its new standards for quality. CalPERS revealed the health plans that scored best and worst in a survey of member satisfaction. Among those at the bottom of the scale were four of the biggest names in the health care industry.

Forced to undergo extensive and tumultuous changes, many players have found it difficult to adapt quickly enough to meet the market's needs and to control their own destinies. They were used to thinking of strategy in material terms: They built new hospital wings, bought fancy new computer networks, installed the latest software panacea, or increased the number of X-ray machines and operating rooms. It is, at best, a stopgap approach to planning production in an industry never short on surprises.

We found many health care leaders, like Larry Gray of FHP California, who ensure the success of their organizations by visualizing strategy not as a thing but as a motion, a continuous activity executed by people who refuse to accept the status quo or to be complacent. We studied all types of health organizations whose leaders engaged in the struggle to construct winning strategies. Our discoveries, we believe, will be useful to other health care organizations as they plan their constructive responses to the forces for change.

# REFERENCES

The Battle for Cleveland. 1994. *Integrated Healthcare Report*, September, 1–8.

Blendon, R., R. Leitman, Ian Morrison, and K. Donelan. 1990. Satisfaction with health systems in ten nations. *Health Affairs 9*, Summer: 185–92.

Ferguson, Tom. 1995. Consumer health informatics. *Healthcare Forum*, January–February, 28–32.

———1995. E-mail medicine. *Wall Street Journal.* February 27.

Jimenez, Ralph. 1995. States consider rating system in Pennsylvania, a consumer can look up providers in book. *Boston Globe,* June 25, 6.

Kiely, Thomas. 1993. The right chemistry. *CIO*, October 15, 37–41.

Koco, Linda. 1994. Oregon Blues offer "kids-only" health insurance plan. *National Underwriter Life & Health*, September 19, 13.

Rauber, Chris. 1994. 21st century vision. *Healthcare Forum*, January–February, 75–78.

United HealthCare Corporation. 1994. Annual report.

Warden, Gail. 1995. Interview with Ken Jennings. November 20.

Winslow, Ron. 1996. Emergency-room visits fall as HMOs target overuse. *Wall Street Journal*, March 7, B2.

Winslow, Ron. 1995. New "Report Card" on health plans uses standardized criteria. *Wall Street Journal*, February 4, B6.

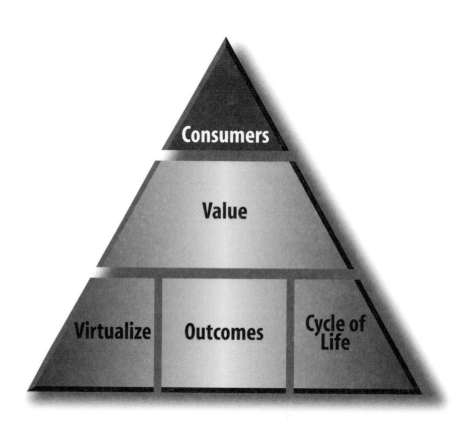

# 2

---

# WINNING STRATEGIES:
# THE VALUE
# FOR CUSTOMERS

---

W hat are the three words on the lips of all customers these days? *Cost. Quality. Service.* No
doubt you hear them every day. These are the
words around which consumer groups rally, pressuring organizations to change their practices and accommodate their demands. Some of your customers, still timid and deferential
around medical specialists, whisper their discontent; others,
thoroughly exasperated with what they see as a hopelessly in-
ept health care system, scream out.

Whatever the volume, it is a safe bet that no health care enterprise can stay around if it does not pay heed. Those organizations that formulate new strategies even as they turn a deaf
ear to consumer cries, and those that dress up their health
care slogans with fancy rhetoric, will soon be talking only to
themselves. From the consumers' point of view, their words
need no translation and abide no euphemisms. They want
value.

Many health care organizations have begun to listen to those demands, responding with products and services that have empirically established outcomes to show their effectiveness. Aetna Professional Management Corporation (APMC), a subsidiary of Aetna, for example, heard its customers' message static-free and answered immediately. According to Scott Cleary and Linda Ronan of Andersen Consulting, this is what happened: After decades as one of the largest indemnity insurers, Aetna determined that it needed to build local care delivery capacity to offer its customers the services of primary care physicians, internists, and nurses. Organized around family practices in nine major geographic areas, this hub-and-spoke health care system will introduce innovative technology to improve services to customers. (Ronan 1995)

APMC is building a computer network that will allow a member who normally works in Los Angeles to receive health care even while on a business trip to Dallas: The member will be able to access APMC data online. A mother, frantic to protect her child from a highly contagious infection, will be able to call into the system and speak to a nurse who has immediate access to the child's records and care protocols. Seamlessly combining the data from medical records, physicians' schedules, insurance payments, and clinical treatments, the planned system will provide—in a matter of seconds rather than hours—a service that saves money for both the member and the system. APMC estimates savings of 25 percent over the traditional ways of treating customers. Hospital emergency rooms will no longer be clogged up with people whose illnesses do not demand immediate treatment; customers will receive higher-quality health care at lower costs; and health care professionals will do their jobs free of the bureaucratic tangles of traditional health care delivery. Indeed, the system APMC is building exemplifies the first strategy we believe every organization needs to develop.

▼ ***Strategy 1:*** Keep ahead of consumers. Innovate continuously to introduce new operating methods, create new services, and provide new products at the level your customers demand.

Only a decade or so ago, it seemed as if there were no limits on what health care organizations and physicians, working on a fee-for-service basis, could charge individuals and their insurers. Hospitals and physicians passed costs (along with a few of their own) to their customers. Meanwhile, a litigious public, looking for any hint of malpractice, aggressively pursued the health care industry, sensing where the riches lay. As a result, costs soared.

Winning organizations, we soon discovered, have a common solution. In an example of bold innovation directed at the consumer, Zeneca Corporation, a pharmaceutical enterprise in Great Britain, purchased hospitals, began operating its own HMO, and established aggressive services for managing disease. Methodist Medical Center of Illinois, a hospital in Peoria, developed a new drug, fludeoxyglucose, and is seeking FDA approval. (Edwards 1995) And Catherine Smith, who heads the strategy and communications group at Aetna Health Plans (AHP), believes that aggressive genetic testing for illnesses such as Alzheimer's will bring AHP directly into new approaches to health. (Smith 1995)

These organizations, and many more like them, are putting together effective strategies to find the right combination of innovative products and services that will spell value for the consumer. They are working to keep the customers they have while reaching out to potential new ones.

Bruce Campbell, a physician executive at Aetna, describes the imperative to control medical costs as one of his organization's three "burning platforms," do-or-die ultimatums that AHP considers critical to its continued success. "If we cannot price competitively," Campbell says, "we aren't even in the game." (Campbell 1995) As part of its vision, Aetna Health Plans merged with US Healthcare to position itself as one of the most efficient providers in terms of costs to members.

Tom Williams, an executive at Aetna Health Plans, also aims to reduce the high costs to members. As part of Aetna's overall strategy to transform itself from a risk-averse, traditional indemnity insurer into a risk-taking health care organization, Williams helped to create an innovative HMO for senior citizens in Southern California in the late 1980s: It offers them advanced medical coverage and a number of other services in specialized managed care—pharmaceutical services, vision care services, and managed dental care.

Williams recounts his innovative plan for Aetna to sponsor receptions for its senior citizens from Southern California. These receptions offer seniors the opportunity to get out of their homes and join at special gatherings where they can socialize while learning about Aetna's services. Williams recalls a health plan "birthday party" in a small California town that drew almost 2,000 senior citizens. By engaging people in such social events, Aetna gained a huge competitive advantage in the market by improving retention in its senior health program. (Williams 1995)

All of these programs seek to innovate in response to consumers' incessant demand for lower costs. To create value for customers, health care managers have turned their attention to finding new ways to reduce costs while continuing to provide quality health care and heading off the slash-and-burn proposals of politicians and others who do not fully appreciate the complexities of the health care market.

Many people fear that cost reduction means lower-quality health care. Indeed, consumers have often heard that the more members an HMO enrolls, the lower the price will be for everyone. The drawback, they believe, is interminable waits to see overworked primary care physicians whose main job is to prevent the members' further progress toward the specialist's office. They assume that primary care physicians are little more than gatekeepers. In their opinion, quality sinks rapidly while costs inch downward.

High quality, however, is not necessarily a result of high spending—as many winning health care organizations illustrate. In the past, patients who suffered heart attacks might remain in the hospital for weeks under constant supervision, toting up astronomical bills. Today, however, such notable institutions as Samaritan Hospital in Lebanon, Pennsylvania, deliver excellent care at lower costs. Utilizing innovative work design, Samaritan reduces the length of patients' hospital stays. A multidisciplinary team of hospital and home care staff coordinates each patient's care, from arrival at the hospital's emergency room through the weeks of recuperation at home. Care team nurses make about 40 percent of the home care visits, educating patients and their families on how to monitor progress. In its first three months of operation, the team reduced the readmission rate from 12 to 3 percent, and it saved the hospital $776,000, much to the delight of CEO Robert Longo, who has extended the care model to other diseases. ("A Patient's Perspective" 1994)

In Spokane, Washington, St. Luke's Rehabilitation Institute now combines the work of two facilities. The two institutions, practically next-door neighbors, had for years been strong competitors. Fourteen managers from the two organizations exchanged ideas in sometimes heated, sometimes congenial meetings. In the course of their discussions, as they sought to cut costs, streamline services, and improve the quality of care, they proposed eliminating some of their own jobs. Now operating under the direction of only three managers,

St. Luke's is a model of innovative case management. ("Two Rehab Programs Merge" 1994)

Similarly, the dialysis center at Kaiser Permanente in Los Angeles enjoys its well-deserved reputation as being among the nation's best, yet it too watches costs. Treating large numbers of diabetics—patients whose mortality rate is among the highest for all dialysis patients—the Kaiser Permanente dialysis center sustains an outstanding record of success: The mortality rate for its patients is only 16 percent, a third less than the national average. In addition, Kaiser Permanente patients spend a third fewer days in the hospital for their treatments. (Eichenwald 1995)

Value-conscious consumers tell us that they are particularly concerned about the quality of their health care. Their demand for quality is a close second to their demand for lower costs. As illustrated by Aetna, St. Luke's Rehabilitation Hospital, and the Kaiser Permanente dialysis center in Los Angeles, high quality need not be eviscerated by cost-cutting proposals. The health care organization that settles for lower quality makes a strategic error: It will be a second-rate institution, or it will fail altogether.

Following lower costs and higher quality, it is easy to see why the third member of the triumvirate of health care demands is better service. Members of HMOs press for more choices and easier access to primary care physicians and specialists. They despise bureaucratic runaround, wasted time spent in waiting rooms, misplaced medical records, and unsatisfactory resolution of disagreements with physicians, hospitals, insurers, and others in the industry. More and more are asking for "one-stop shopping" and a seamless care experience.

In response to these demands, health care organizations are exploring a myriad of tools and services to enable such seamless care. These tools span a broad range of processes, from collecting detailed information about individual consumers in order to tailor and customize the care experience through sophisticated information management systems that allow information to be shared across organizational boundaries and care to be coordinated in a more seamless manner. For example, tools such as health risk appraisals can provide a wealth of information about individual health care needs, issues, and preferences. This information can then be used to guide the development, implementation, and monitoring of longitudinal care paths or customer service plans.

The organizations that anticipate consumers' demands and respond most effectively to their calls for change are best positioned to succeed in the future. St. Vincent's Hospital of Melbourne, Australia, for example, has found a way to reduce the average length of hospital stays. By expanding its ambulatory and community services program, St. Vincent's can focus on those who require home health care for chronic diseases and disabilities. Rather than waiting for 60-odd state and federal agencies to agree on how to fund this continuum of care, St. Vincent's executives undertook a three-year change program and redesigned every care path, job, and business process. Guided by demographic data that showed an aging population living in the inner city, far from the hospital facility, St. Vincent's leaders agreed that its large stand-alone hospital would quickly become a dinosaur. Accordingly, the change management team recommended installing an extensive network to allow the free flow of medical information among health care professionals and customers wherever and whenever they need it.

Equally concerned with creating innovations for the customer, Walter S. Becker, the CEO of Medina Memorial Hospital, saw the advantages of partnering with the community. A small regional institution near Buffalo, New York, Medina

Memorial has seen its financial picture improve dramatically in the last few years. In both 1992 and 1993, the hospital announced net incomes of $850,000—an improvement in the bottom line that Becker attributes largely to Community Partners, its outreach program. Targeting the poor and the uninsured, the hospital has established a prenatal care center that provides valuable clinical services and education to the community, which includes large numbers of pregnant teens and people with histories of abusing or neglecting their children. (Rauber 1994: 76–77)

Even such giant companies as Baxter International, Johnson & Johnson, Eli Lilly, Searle, and Merck are expanding their services beyond merely providing drugs and medical products to offering direct and extensive health care. Saul Kaplan, managing partner, Pharmaceutical and Medical Products of Andersen Consulting, believes that many of the major pharmaceutical and health products companies are remarkably well positioned to take advantage of this service market. Pharmaceutical and health products organizations are now mobilizing to innovate in the complex system of health care professionals, organizations, government agencies, service providers, and customers.

Cardinal Health, a traditional pharmaceutical distributor in Dublin, Ohio, recently decided to extend value to customers by offering simple diagnostic procedures through its "Medicine Shoppe" facilities in selected locations. Now instead of simply filling prescriptions, Cardinal Health provides tests for blood pressure, glucose levels, diabetes, and other conditions, thereby building in extra value for customers.

Given the surging demand for alternative medicine that involves meditation and biofeedback, Sharp HealthCare of San Diego, California, opened its Institute for Human Potential and Mind/Body Medicine in 1993. The institute teaches patients both Western preventive-medicine practices of relaxation, exercise, and diet, as well as principles and practices from India, such as meditation and yoga. The institute is even conducting clinical trials on groups of patients to assess the efficacy of its preventive-medicine treatments compared with traditional ones. (Hagland et al. 1995: 84)

In their effort to anticipate the consumer's needs—often before the consumer recognizes them—these health care organizations illustrate how they incorporate the first strategy into their new market positions. The essence of this strategy is their willingness to take risks: They are expanding services, looking for innovative ways to cut costs, and improving the quality of care delivery. Those organizations are putting into practice the theoretical observations that Gary Hamel and C.K. Prahalad offer in their study of strategic intent; that is, as they launch new businesses and provide startling new value for consumers, those organizations are "creating tomorrow's competitive advantages faster than competitors [can copy them]." (Hamel and Prahalad 1989: 69)

▼ ***Strategy 2:*** Cut to the moment of value by eliminating middlemen, dead time, unnecessary steps—anyone or anything that does not add value. Bring care directly to consumers through interactive technology.

Counting all the hours spent making an appointment, getting to the doctor's office, filling out forms, and reading old magazines in the waiting room, the average consumer wastes about 90 percent of time allocated to health care on what we call non-value-added activities. For what is often no more than a few minutes of face-to-face discussion with a physician, a patient or a member of an HMO can lose half a day from work

*Figure 7* Winning Strategies

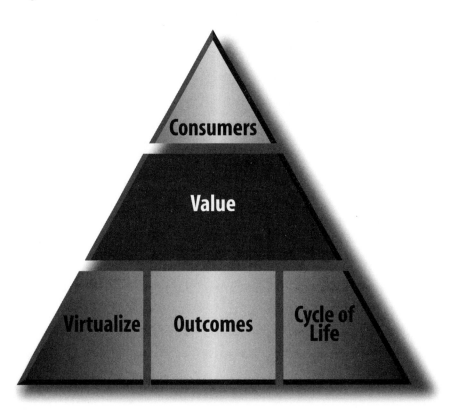

and family. No other consumer-dependent industry requires such commitment and exacts such a toll.

Why is it important to cut to the moment of value by removing health care's barriers and middlemen? It is obvious that streamlined processes are more efficient and save customers money and time, but there is a more practical answer: If your organization forces customers to endure such inconveniences and fails to humanize its contact with them, the customers will exercise their choice and move elsewhere.

Today's health care industry is adopting innovative processes and systems that bring the customer to the moment of value. In an exciting venture to streamline and digitize the delivery of health care, a consortium that includes the Walt Disney Company, the Adventist Health System, Florida Hospital, and two subsidiaries of Eli Lilly is planning the construction of Celebration City, a new community near Orlando, Florida. There, comprehensive health care services will soon be available to more than 20,000 senior citizens. Each home will come equipped with a computer and other telecommunication devices to give residents instant access to Celebration Health, the organization that will coordinate a primary care team for each resident. Members will also have access to the staff of local hospitals, pharmacists, home health care providers, insurers, and a rich network of accessible and user-friendly medical information.

By design, Celebration City will bring health care directly to consumers, eliminating many of the time-consuming barriers to today's health care systems, whether located in New York, New Delhi, or New South Wales. When Celebration City residents undergo standard diagnostic tests—finger sticks, electrocardiograms, or urine analyses, for example—the results will be available to them as well as their care providers through Internet connections and on-site connection points, eventually, perhaps, without even having to leave their homes. Primary care teams will manage the seniors' preventive care in a manner akin to the archaic but much-loved practice of daily house calls. Those calls, however, will be virtual house calls, made possible by the wonders of information technology and telecommunications.

Similar in structure and services, Friendly Hills in La Habra, California, offers an entire health care network to 16,000 senior citizens. Simply by calling in questions or searching online, any resident can receive an education in wellness and self-monitored health care. Those who have recently undergone hip replacement surgery, for example, have a chance to learn how to walk on crutches, how to lose weight, and how to hasten their progress back to good health. The service tracks calls and monitors treatments, and it discourages residents from rushing to the emergency room or the doctor's office with insignificant ailments. ("Is Friendly Hills" 1994: 30) The Friendly Hills network takes full responsibility for the care of all 16,000 seniors, including measures for preventing illness and injury. Gloria Mayer, the president of Friendly Hills, expresses the organization's philosophy best when she says, "If you wait until the patient comes to the hospital, you've waited too long. We see hospitalization as a failure of the system." (Qtd. in Lumsdon 1995: 82)

No less impressive is On Lok, an HMO founded 12 years ago by senior citizens in San Francisco's Chinatown. On Lok, which means "happy, peaceful abode," provides care delivery at a day center where seniors meet with their doctors, nurses, therapists, pharmacists, social workers, and financial advisers. The convenience that On Lok offers its members is unsurpassed, particularly for the elderly who often lack the mobility or the transportation to get to distant clinics and specialists. Indeed, On Lok's service has become so popular that it has recently expanded to ten other cities and has plans for future extensions. (Hagland et al. 1995: 90)

If it is true that what starts in California quickly spreads to the rest of the country, we can look forward to many more such communities. Senior citizens will be among the first to benefit. Residents in retirement villages or self-contained communities will have computer networks that can put them directly in touch with their care givers and transmit complex medical data such as MRI scans, patient records, and treatment protocols. Initial forays into this area are proving so popular that other organizations will soon recognize the potential benefits of offering those services on an even larger scale.

While no one will claim that every member's frustrating experiences with health care providers will suddenly evaporate, we can look forward to more fully integrated and efficient care delivery. Putting our second strategy at the top of their agenda, organizations that cut to the moment of value will find that by eliminating bureaucratic layers and other non-value-adding steps, they can help direct their products and services to the people who most need care.

If they are slow to adopt this strategy on their own, health care organizations will likely find that consumer groups will prod them to change. The Buyers Health Care Action Group (BHCAG) in Minneapolis, for example, represents several important consumer groups in Minnesota, including the large and powerful coalition of state employees. Rather than allowing middlemen to negotiate the prices of health care, the Buyers Group contracts directly with doctors and hospitals, bypassing several layers of intermediaries.

While groups like BHCAG are instrumental in eliminating some of the administrative complexity in the health care industry, an even more powerful force for change is technology: Computer networks, teleconferencing, the Internet, and health information services now speed medical information practically anywhere in the world, wherever there are transmitters and receivers, mechanical or human. Already, for instance, a physician in Oklahoma or Saudi Arabia can send a patient's X-rays to specialists at the Mayo Clinic in Minnesota or the Cleveland Clinic in Ohio. The specialists, in turn, study the images and offer interpretations of the patient's condition. Second opinions are just a mouse click away. A radiologist at a cost-troubled facility may see his job eliminated when a new virtual radiology job opens up with an organization that specializes in distance medicine. Although painful, the health care industry will see a shifting of employees that is similar to the shifts we now see in banking, manufacturing, and communications.

The patients of the future may well meet a virtual doctor through the same computer network that now provides them with copious medical information. (Scott 1994) The opportunities are limitless, and many Internet services already offer health information sources similar to America's House Call (AHC) Network. Developed by Orbis Broadcast Group, AHC allows subscribers to locate information about specific diseases or conditions, to ask questions of health care professionals, and to correspond with support groups and referral services about possible drug therapies, surgeries, and effects of medication. (PRNewswire 1995) Because companies must deal with a plethora of information available in easily accessible forms, they face the daunting job of interpreting the data, understanding the risks of certain treatments, and measuring the quality of that information. Therefore, just as software programs for preparing tax returns are not likely to replace actual accountants, online medical services will not substitute for physicians, nurses, and other care givers. In fact, health care professionals may find their services in greater demand once customers begin educating themselves about their medical conditions.

Future physicians, in fact, may be pleasantly surprised at just how knowledgeable their patients are, once they have access to medical data on disease management. Invariably, there will be some consumers who will misunderstand that data or insist on inappropriate drug therapies, but others will find that the information empowers them to ask the right questions and to challenge the cost of medical procedures.

Health care organizations that adopt a strategy to eliminate non-value-adding processes will no doubt encounter widespread resistance. No one wants to be thought of as having nothing of value to contribute. Certainly there will be few individuals as courageous as those Spokane, Washington, executives who approved plans to eliminate certain of their own jobs. Enterprises that adopt bold strategies need to determine—to everyone's satisfaction and clear understanding—how their strategies will provide value and how each employee, business process, and partner contributes to that value.

Health care executives must now ask hard questions about value: For whom or for what does each process or job have value? What's valuable to the hospital as a business enterprise may not have value for the patients who use its services. Regina Herzlinger, a professor of business administration at Harvard Business School, recounts a personal experience that illustrates that distinction: When she called a hospital to report an error in billing, a hospital administrator inquired why she had bothered. After all, an insurance company was actually paying the bill. (Herzlinger 1994: 89) That anecdote underscores the central issue that all players—care givers, insurers, providers, administrators, patients, and members themselves—must recognize their collective responsibility in defining and ensuring value throughout the industry.

In this era of ready information exchange, customers are educating themselves on what constitutes value. Their scrutiny of the very same criteria health care organizations themselves use puts them in a good position to evaluate products, outcomes, and health care delivery. Many consumers, for example, understand and can explain analytic differences between Prozac and Zoloft. (Langreth 1996) They are just as likely to judge physicians, HMOs, and hospitals by empirical data as by reputation. It is no longer unusual, for instance, for consumers to research the mortality rates of dialysis centers before entrusting their lives to one.

In short, health care professionals can demonstrate their

receptiveness to consumer demand for lower costs, higher quality, and better service by anticipating demands and eliminating processes that add no value to the delivery of care. Winning organizations create unprecedented value by bringing care and products directly to the consumer through technology and new business ventures designed not just to cure sickness but to keep people healthy.

In the next chapter, we examine three other strategies that health care organizations need to implement to set the best value in products, outcomes, and delivery. As they chart the courses for their organizations to follow, executives will find inspiration and illumination in the successes (and failures) of other health care enterprises.

# REFERENCES

Campbell, Bruce. 1995. Interview with Ken Jennings and Sharyn Materna. May.

Edwards, Nicholas. 1995. Pharmaceutical industry responses to managed care. Presentation at the Conference on European Pharmaceutical Companies in Managed Care. October.

Eichenwald, Kurt. 1995. Making incentives work in kidney patients' favor. *New York Times*, December 6, B1, B15.

Hagland, Mark, et al. 1995. The cutting edge: technology, places, people. *Hospitals & Health Networks*, August 5, 79ff.

Hamel, Gary, and C. K. Prahalad. 1989. Strategic intent. *Harvard Business Review* 67 (May–June): 63–76.

Herzlinger, Regina. 1994. The quiet health care revolution. *The Public Interest*, No. 115 (Spring): 72–90.

Is Friendly Hills where we're headed? 1994. *Hospitals & Health Networks*, November 20, 30.

Langreth, Robert. 1996. High anxiety: rivals threaten Prozac's reign. *Wall Street Journal*, May 9, B1, B3.

Lumsdon, Kevin. 1995. Friendly Hills HealthCare Network. *Hospitals & Health Networks*, August 5: 82.

A patient's perspective. 1994. *Hospitals & Health Networks*, November 20, 38.

PRNewswire (Chicago). 1995. [Orbis Broadcast Group]. June 21.

Rauber, Chris. 1994. Communities that are making a difference. *Healthcare Forum*, July–August, 73–77.

Ronan, Linda. 1995. Interview with Susan Vanderpool. Hartford, Conn.

Scott, Lisa. 1994. Will healthcare accept the "virtual" doctor? *Modern Healthcare*, November 28, 34–35, 38, 40–42.

Smith, Catherine. 1995. Interview with Susan Vanderpool and Tom Dunne.

Two rehab programs merge. 1994. *Hospitals & Health Networks*, November 20, 36.

Williams, Thomas R. 1995. Interview with Sharyn Materna and Ken Jennings.

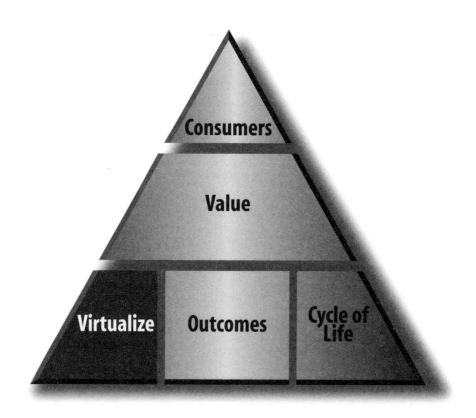

# 3

## WINNING STRATEGIES: PRODUCTS, OUTCOMES, DELIVERIES

A t 6:30 a.m., two Minneapolis paramedics answered an elderly woman's call to 911. Deftly maneuvering their ambulance through morning traffic, they arrived 20 minutes later and found her sitting on her kitchen floor surrounded by boxes, overturned furniture, and a dozen broken eggs. A quick check of her vital signs revealed only a slightly elevated pulse—nothing more than a mild case of anxiety. She was disoriented and confused but fortunately had no broken bones.

This woman, the paramedics determined, really had no need of an ambulance. Living in a cluttered, dirty house, she hobbled from kitchen to bathroom to bedroom and back, negotiating an obstacle course, which on that day had caused her to drop the carton of eggs as she prepared her breakfast. The next day or the day after, that clutter might make her ill from poor hygiene or cause her to fall and break a hip.

In the midst of that disarray, one of the paramedics spied a Medica Health Plans (a health plan owned by Allina) card and decided to call. That afternoon, an Allina representative and a social worker arranged to have the house cleaned and inspected for safety hazards. Later, home care givers installed support rails in the bathroom, removed boxes and furniture from the woman's path, and assisted her in planning a nutritious diet. Although the initial emergency call was technically a false alarm, the paramedics had issued an alarm of their own: They took the initiative to correct the situation before it became a major problem, setting in motion a course of action that would bring together numerous health care professionals. Drawing on the best practices of many health care organizations, the care givers joined in an effort to restore the woman to better health and to help her avoid future illnesses and calamities. Since then, she has stayed out of the local hospital emergency room and is living a much healthier life.

"That story needs to be repeated a million times," says David Strand, a vice president at Allina Health System in Minneapolis. "Suddenly, you have the whole system working to create an environment for people where they can be healthier." (Strand 1995)

But it might just as well be a story that illustrates the kinds of change necessary throughout the entire health care industry, for it depicts the three winning strategies that we discuss in this chapter. As we saw in the previous chapter, the health care enterprises of the future must adopt strategies that seek to provide greater customer value by continuously innovating to create new services and eliminating non-value-adding services. At the same time, health care managers need to develop three other strategies around products, outcomes, and delivery.

As the two Minneapolis paramedics' performance illustrates, care givers are redefining health care. Curing illnesses is no longer the primary focus of health care. Instead, care givers are looking for innovative ways to mind the full cycle of life and provide a continuum of care for all citizens. No one person, no one health care organization can accomplish this task alone. By working together, however, health care professionals can—and must—stop viewing other organizations as cutthroat competitors and start working in cooperative ventures.

Pursuing a strategy of prevention means that health care enterprises must greatly expand offerings to include immunizations, inexpensive counseling, and screening for such common problems as cancer, hypertension, and heart disease. They must increasingly work with local employers to institute workplace wellness programs that encourage employees to take better care of their health by eating the right foods, dieting, and exercising. A number of organizations (see Chapter 5), for example, are beginning to employ next-generation life care plans that provide for preventive and primary care, episodic interventions, chronic disease management, and overall health and wellness. Still others will provide such services as home inspections and counseling to address the underlying social causes of illness and injury. A few preventive steps, like home inspections, cost far less than an ambulance call and a hospital stay.

▼ *Strategy 3:* Give your best; virtualize the rest. Determine which services and products you can deliver to value-conscious customers and use alliances with the best partners and service suppliers to offer seamless access to the continuum of care.

One of the attitudes that is hardest to overcome is the Atlas complex, named for the mythological giant who had the unenviable task of balancing the world on his shoulders. Many health care managers feel responsible for making their orga-

nizations serve as all things to all people. To liberate themselves from this burden, managers of future health care enterprises will conduct honest appraisals of the resources, talents,
and purposes of their organizations: What are their capacities
and competencies? Can they offer products and services most
efficiently and profitably?

## Vertical Integration Versus Virtual Integration

The significance of our third strategy is most apparent in the
context of the evolving health care industry. On the one hand,
we see many organizations moving toward vertical integration,
through mergers and acquisitions, to expand their capacities
to meet consumer demand or to create new competitive
space. Aetna's $9 billion acquisition of U.S. Healthcare is just
one of many recent and highly publicized examples, and its
success ultimately hinges on integrating the processes, objectives, strategies, and people from both sides. Ron Compton,
CEO of the newly merged entity, sees the advantages of bringing together two highly compatible organizations to provide
better services and products. Handling more than 90 million
claim checks in 1995, Aetna constitutes one of the world's
largest databases of claims payment information. Through the
merger, Aetna gained U.S. Healthcare's expertise in providing
quality treatment and clinical information, as well as unparalleled capability in retail sales. (Compton 1996) Starting with
more than 200,000 providers and 2,300 hospitals, the new
entity emerging has been hailed as an event of seismic pro-
portion in the health care world.

On the other hand, not every organization is ready or eager to merge. Many actively resist acquisition—and we have
seen plenty of instances in other industries banking, telecommunications, and the like—where the acquired company ends

up dysfunctional or the whole deal goes sour. We believe that virtually integrated organizations will become more prevalent than mergers and acquisitions. Two or more organizations are virtually integrated when they form an alliance or partnership based on shared information and incentives. PacifiCare Health Systems, Inc., in Cypress, California, for example, contracts with physician groups and other providers to offer services that it alone could never supply. Not only are virtually integrated organizations less costly than mergers to establish, they also offer the advantage of enabling each organization to focus on continually improving a selected set of core competencies rather than having to be all things to all people. For value-conscious customers, the enormous sums paid to acquire an organization mean very little if the quality and service are not readily available.

Virtually integrated organizations are extremely flexible and protean, assuming many shapes. In the nation's capital, four organizations—Aetna Health Plans of the Mid-Atlantic, Inc.; CapitalCare, a subsidiary of Blue Cross and Blue Shield of the National Capital Area; Chartered Health Plan, a state-approved HMO; and the George Washington University Health Plan—jointly offer FirstHelp, an assessment and referral service patients can access simply by calling a toll-free number. The system design provides for collection of patient data, quick identification of serious medical problems, immediate responses to caller inquiries, and referral to one or more of 3,700 providers at Chartered or 2,000 private-practice physicians associated with the GW Medical Center. ("Four Competing D.C. Health Plans" 1995)

Among the leaders in physician practice management companies (PPMs), MedPartners, Inc., in Birmingham, Alabama, acquired Mullikin Medical Enterprises of Long Beach, California, and recently announced the acquisition of Care-

Mark. The new health care enterprise has projected annual revenues of more than $4 billion. As part of their competitive advantage, PPMs can sell medical services to HMOs for a fixed price while benefiting physicians by contracting with other providers and taking care of administrative tasks such as billing and scheduling, thereby increasing value for the consumer. (Hayes and Rudnitsky 1995)

Recognizing the potential for saving their customers a great deal of money, the health care unit of Cigna Corporation recently announced that it would contract with Smith-Kline Beecham PLC to provide laboratory tests for Cigna Health Care's members. According to the agreement, Cigna will pay SmithKline Beecham a flat rate based on the total number of Cigna members in the plan. The two companies will share information from those test results in a consolidated database, and health care professionals will have access to the data for managing such conditions as high blood pressure and heart disease. (Winslow 1995)

The examples suggest that the future of health care is ideally in partnerships to provide true continuum-of-care programs for their members: family care that extends from birth to death. More and more, we see health care enterprises contracting with other organizations to provide radiology services or home care. Given the complexity of today's medical problems, health care organizations realize that they must outsource; they must form alliances, partnerships, and collaborative ventures. They are, in effect, creating virtual enterprises of extended services for all members.

Mickey Herbert, CEO of Physicians Health Services (PHS) in Trumbull, Connecticut, restates our third strategy this way: "At PHS, we determined that we should become a master contractor rather than a master owner." Herbert built PHS from scratch, intent upon finding practical ways to realize those values he holds more important: providing the highest-quality service and doing what is right for the customer. Between August 1994 and April 1995, Herbert led PHS's expansion into the managed care market of New York, signing up 67 hospitals and 7,500 physicians while establishing a key partnership with the Guardian Insurance Company and its more than 1,000 brokers. (Herbert 1995)

Reflecting on the changing health care environment, Gordon Sprenger, the CEO of Allina Health System, observes that the industry is moving away from strictly competitive relationships. Even now, Allina, a $2-billion not-for-profit managed care organization, occasionally competes with organizations with which it collaborates and cooperates at other times. In the future, however, "competitors and collaborators may be the same," Sprenger predicts. A showpiece for its integrated delivery system, Allina has begun uniting people from various areas who had long perceived each other as competitors. "Our whole game plan," Sprenger says, "was to break down the adversarial relationships that have developed between the financing and the delivery sides of our business." (Sprenger 1995)

*Strategy 3*—give your best; virtualize the rest—focuses attention on products and services. It offers health care managers the opportunity to construct a vision for their organizations—not as isolated, stand-alone corporations fighting off attackers from every side but as integral parts of a community of care providers offering the best services and products to their customers.

The alternatives to cooperation and collaboration are painful and destructive, for they pit one organization against another in a quasi-Darwinian contest where only the fittest survive. The vast changes taking place in health care, however, have radically altered our traditional definitions of fittest: No longer do we extol the largest, the richest, the most politically powerful, or the most diverse. Indeed, the postulates of Darwinian evolution do not apply to the complex world of health care on the brink of the 21st century. We must consider other strategies to plot our future courses.

▼ *Strategy 4:* Mine the riches of outcomes. Capture data on the best practices (those that create the greatest value for customers) and look for opportunities to improve processes to increase that value.

Most health care organizations are treasure troves of both clinical and nonclinical data scattered in patient records, physicians' summaries, financial records, family histories, and

*Figure 8* WINNING STRATEGIES

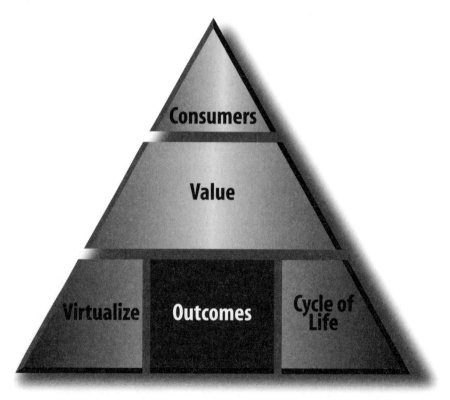

innumerable other sources. Most of the data, however, exists in raw form: It is not yet usable information. We cannot call it knowledge until it has been organized and studied in light of outcomes.

Organizations throughout the industry are developing various measures of outcomes according to such criteria as relative costs, degree of member satisfaction, mortality rates, and the like. Kaiser Permanente's Northern California Region (which we will examine in more detail in Chapter 5) has developed an extensive report card to evaluate its performance. It measures both the effectiveness and the appropriateness of intervention in treating illness. It does so with the conviction that Kaiser Permanente members want to know what value they are getting for their health care dollars. As more and more organizations follow Kaiser Permanente's example, we will have a rich lode of material from which to mine the best practices that produce the greatest value for customers.

At Intermountain Health Care in Salt Lake City, Utah, researchers are already mining the hospital chain's treasures. They have catalogued data from more than 15,000 patients and entered much of it into a database from which they hope to retrieve essential information about the most effective treatments. Intermountain's HELP system, as the database is called, will allow caregivers access to the data, to transform it into information that can be used to create new knowledge: namely, the best treatments, as well as preventive regimens to avoid relapses and recidivism. (Highland et al. 1995: 100)

In a similar effort, the Group Health Cooperative (GHC) of Puget Sound, Washington, is looking at ways to help physicians identify current practices and measure them against optimal ones.

Citing studies recently published in the *New England Journal of Medicine* and the *Journal of the American Medical Association,*

Handley and Stuart note that the GHC strategy is to inform physicians that "a significant percentage of medical practices are ineffective and some may actually be harmful." (Handley and Stuart 1994: 10) Whereas most organizations still rely on the subjective measure of the clinicians' expertise, measured variously in terms of number of papers published, number of operations performed, number of patients treated and read-mitted for the same complaint, GHC of Puget Sound seeks now to provide its physicians and other care givers with solid data. Again, the chief beneficiary is the consumer, whose in-vestment in the corporation rises significantly.

In metropolitan New York City, Aetna members benefit from a recent agreement with Olsten Kimberly QualityCare to collect data from Information Warehouse, "the industry's largest patient database." (Olsten 1995) Having merged with US Healthcare, Aetna is one of the nation's largest managed care organizations. Data collected from its millions of mem-bers of managed care plans provides extraordinarily useful in-formation on specific outcomes.

As Aetna Chairman and CEO Ron Compton notes, a wealth of information about outcomes enables the company to focus on its best practices, which, in turn, benefits its cus-tomers and members. In our interview, Compton recounted watching the U.S. Healthcare videotape of a two-day workshop in which twelve of the best hip-replacement surgeons in the country met to discuss the most effective treatments and pro-cedures. The videotaped meeting was transferred to CD-ROM and sent to health care providers. That session on hip re-placements is only one of thirty procedures that have been videotaped. (Compton 1996)

In Palo Alto, California, the Veterans' Administration Medical Center is compiling a large database that details re-sults of patients' treatments. That information will be available to other care givers, many of whom are thousands of miles from Palo Alto. Guided by Adam Siever, a physician at the Stanford University Medical Center, the VA began installing an electronic charting system in its surgical intensive care unit. Later, it added a similar system for its medical ICU. In addition to bedside monitoring, these systems collect and organize data that researchers and health care professionals use to evaluate treatments.

New Internet-based capabilities, accessible by far-flung health care organizations, allow for the creation of diverse virtually merged databases that provide extraordinarily large samples for the study of particular diseases and disorders. Managed care organizations, providers, pharmaceutical companies, and others are all investing significant time and resources in this area. The trend will grow as clinicians and health care managers look for aggregated data to improve clinical processes and thereby increase value for consumers.

▼ ***Strategy 5:*** Mind the cycle of life. Design and market health care products and services that create consumer value by preventing illness, enhancing health, and easing the debilitating effects of chronic disease.

The story goes that in China you stop paying your doctor when you get sick. Whether or not that is true today, before long it may well be the case in many other countries. Whereas traditional medical approaches are designed to detect, treat, and cure diseases, future health care programs will focus on prevention measures and interventions. Cancer, cardiovascular disease, and other devastating illnesses have long been the subjects of early screening programs. Many of those tests are expensive, and observers have pointed out the tests don't guarantee good health. There is little evidence that mammography tests for women under 50, for example, can be jus-

*Figure 9* WINNING STRATEGIES

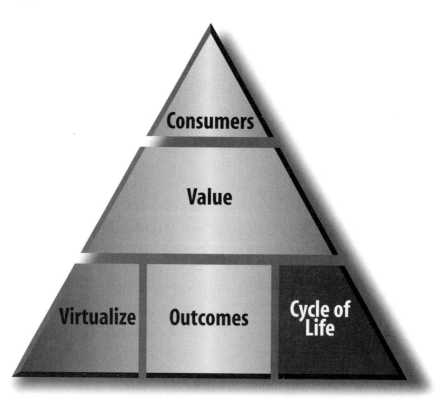

tified. The sad truth is that prevention measures by themselves can neither keep mortality at bay nor hold the lid on increasing medical costs. (Leutwyler 1995: 127, 129; Green et al. 1992)

Nevertheless, there is growing evidence that health care organizations should invest heavily in targeted preventive care and wellness programs. Companies that offer their employees the chance to exercise daily or to enroll in diet-control and smoking-cessation programs realize as much as a 20-percent reduction in their medical expenses. (Leutwyler 1995: 125) Hackley Hospital in Muskegon, Michigan, for example, has opened profitable outpatient centers where local residents can learn about prenatal health care and wellness programs that have immediate relevance, especially for people who live in the inner city. (Rauber 1994: 76)

### Telephone and Internet Advice Services

Among the most popular and innovative programs encouraging the public to take a greater interest in promoting its own health is a toll-free phone service that initially puts callers in touch with a registered nurse who answers questions, makes references or recommendations, and provides information to help allay callers' fears. Aetna's Tom Williams helped develop Informed Health, a self-care program that connects callers to a specialty nurse who offers medical advice and counseling. "If you give people information and engage them in self-care, they begin to act as providers of their own health care," Williams says, "and they will become more efficient utilizers of health care resources. They become more actively involved in managing their own care and better patients since they know what questions to ask their physician, and they feel more confident in asking. Informed Health actually empowers them to take these initiatives." (Williams 1995)

Services such as Informed Health are taking the market by storm. For less than $6 a month, consumers can purchase a membership in "Tele-Dr.," a service provided by Medical Consultants of America, Inc., which allows customers to use a new 800 number to receive advice and information from physicians. ("New 800" 1994) "Personal Health Advisor," or PHA, is one of the services that Access Health provides to other organizations such as Blue Cross of Western Pennsylvania. It educates people to take better care of themselves, to make what Joy Gaetano, project manager of PHA, calls "smart decisions" about their health. (Barnet 1995).

"Electronic" doctors are available 24 hours a day on the Internet. Whatever ails you—arthritis, osteoporosis, cancer, HIV infection—help is just a mouse click away. (Briley 1993; Ransom 1993; Wolff 1995) Healthcare Data Information Corporation (HDIC), a nonprofit consortium of some of California's largest hospitals, HMOs, and other providers, links customers and various community health information networks (CHINs) into a super network that is projected to save up to $3 billion annually. (Borzo 1995)

Health care professionals continue to debate the usefulness and accuracy of information given out by toll-free services and on Internet bulletin boards and chat rooms. (Roan 1995) Still, there is abundant evidence that consumers are willing to pay to satisfy their craving for information and advice about health-related issues. If highly respected and reliable organizations do not answer this need, you can bet there are others more than willing to go into that potentially lucrative market.

## Community-Based Health Programs

What works for individuals can also work for entire communities. A study of one community's hospital revealed that the seven most common reasons for emergency room visits were (in order of frequency) automobile accidents, personal attacks, accidents not involving automobiles, bronchial ailments, alcoholism, drug-related problems, and dog bites. (McKnight 1994: 41) Although from one point of view, health care professionals must deal with the people who present themselves for treatment, regardless of where or how they received their injuries, those caregivers are also aware that many emergency cases are social problems.

Around the country, health care organizations are working to address these medical problems, whatever their ultimate source. TMCare in Tucson, Arizona, for instance, has created a program where former competitors now collaborate in an effort to improve immunizations for children in the community. In addition, it will run twenty-six preventive health care clinics in area schools, particularly in the poorer areas of the city. Reflecting the attitude of many health care executives, Hank Walker, the CEO of TMCare, says that "the ultimate measures of our success are the health indexes of our community."(Heilig 1994: 77)

Similar preventive community-health programs have appeared in many other cities. In Columbus, Ohio, a fully equipped van owned by U.S. Health Corporation parks at two inner-city high schools to offer free prenatal services to students. A six-person team offers pregnancy tests, postpartum care, and counseling on the use of drugs and alcohol.

Miracle Village in Cleveland offers women addicted to drugs and alcohol a three-month live-in program of counseling and treatment. Operated by the MetroHealth Medical Center, the village houses 30 families—mothers and their children—whom it helps to keep out of trauma units and foster homes. (Hudson 1995)

In Baltimore, the Johns Hopkins Hospital has joined with a group of community religious leaders to institute a program called Heart, Body, and Soul. It seeks to address some of the most demanding social problems affecting people's health: drug addiction, violence, poor diet, and poverty. Staffed by volunteers and sponsored by a cross-section of civic, government, and business groups, Heart, Body, and Soul has launched initiatives that include health screening programs, prevention centers, and medical counseling and treatment clinics. In addition, the program founders have "established community crime patrols, crime prevention and education workshops, and housing, education, and economic development programs." (Sasenick 1994: 8)

Each of those community projects operates under the premise that minding the cycle of life requires a wider vision of health than the traditional hospital's view. The web of society reaches beyond the symbolic walls dividing rich from poor, privileged from destitute, even healthy from unhealthy. As we will see in Chapter 6, one of the most successful and innovative organizations, the Henry Ford Health Care System, has for years led the way in providing quality health care to residents of Detroit, and it has not hesitated to extend its services to those areas that other health care facilities have shunned.

Our fifth strategy, minding the cycle of life, focuses attention on the delivery of health care, wherever it is needed. This strategy embodies a strong sense of obligation to enhance the health of all citizens, not just those who are sick and in need of care. Therefore, it expands the definitions of cost, quality, and service, the three words that are most important to our customers.

The five strategies we propose accomplish a number of market shifts. Health care organizations must recognize and prepare for them. As represented in Figure 10, the shifts indicate what we believe to be the transition from the health care industry of the past to that of the future. By innovating continuously, developing new products and services, and launching new businesses that provide unprecedented value for customers, health enterprises can take advantage of the palpable shifts in emphasis that we feel in the industry today. Whereas in the past, the focus was clearly on the physician, the hospital, the research institution, today that is no longer true. The consumer is cracking the whip, demanding value in every aspect of health care.

The health care organization of the past operated under a heavy bureaucracy with numerous middlemen and processes to erect barriers to customers. The enterprise of the future, we

***Figure 10*** MARKET SHIFTS

| Health Care Organization | PAST | FUTURE |
|---|---|---|
| Orientation | Provider-focused | Customer-focused |
| Strategies | Quality at any price | Lower costs, higher quality, and better service |
| Business structure | Hierarchical management, strong sense of bureaucracy | Partnerships and alliances for outsourcing |
| Operating methods | Traditional and static | Innovative new businesses, products, and services |
| Control of information | Restricted to the medical profession | Accessible by individuals and communities |
| Medical objectives | Treatment and cure of diseases and illnesses | Treatment and cure of diseases, early detection and intervention, and prevention and wellness programs |
| Time of treatment | Moment that illness is detected | Continuum-of-care treatment and advice |

believe, will seek to eliminate those non-value-adding elements and to establish long-term partnerships with organizations that offer services for increased value to customers. Many of those services will be virtual, relying on advanced information technology, and many will address health issues throughout an individual's life rather than at the moment of diagnosis or detection.

Processes, reengineered to reflect the longitudinal maintenance of health (physical, mental, and spiritual), will provide a rich source of information about best practices and outcomes. The health enterprises that capture and convert the data into practical solutions will be the future's winners.

The five strategies depend, however, on the health organization's competencies to support, develop, and pursue them. Many people believe it is an indisputable maxim that previous success is no guarantee of future success. Accordingly, we hold that organizations need to examine themselves closely for four fundamental competencies: liberating the consumer, managing individual and population health, delivering excellence in service, and aligning services and resources. It is to those four competencies that we turn in the second part of our vision for future health care.

# References

Barnet, Alicia Ault. 1995. Is knowledge really power for patients? *Business & Health* 13 (May): 29.

Borzo, Greg. 1995. Largest health information network powers up in California. *American Medical News*, September 18, 10.

Briley, Michael. 1993. Arthritis relief—by phone. *Arthritis Today* 7 (November– December): 8.

Compton, Ron. 1996. Interview with the authors. April 18.

Four competing D.C. health plans form historic association. 1995. September 28. PRNewswire.

Handley, Matthew R., and Michael E. Stuart. 1994. An evidence-based approach to evaluating and improving clinical practice: guideline development. *HMO Practice* 8.1 (March 11): 10–19.

Hayes, John R., and Howard Rudnitsky. 1995. M.D. Inc. *Forbes*, September 11, 222–227.

Heilig, Steve. 1994. A visit with the Healthcare Forum's incoming chair: Hank Walker. *Healthcare Forum*, May–June, 76–79.

Herbert, Mickey. 1995. Interview with Ken Jennings. Hartford, Conn. October 17.

Highland, Mark, et al. 1995. The cutting edge: technology, places, people. *Hospitals & Health Networks*, August 5, 79ff.

Hudson, Terese. 1995. MetroHealth Medical Center. *Hospitals & Health Networks*, April 20, 34–35.

Hudson, Terese. 1988. MetroHealth Medical Center. *Hospitals & Health Networks*, April 20, 34, 35.

Leutwyler, Kristin. 1995. The price of prevention. *Scientific American*, April, 124-29.

McKnight, John L. 1994. Hospitals and the health of their communities. *Hospitals & Health Networks*, January 5, 40–41.

New 800 telephone service offers unlimited advice, information from physicians. 1994. PRNewswire, Feb. 28.

Olsten Kimberly. 1995. QualityCare and Aetna Health Plans sign major agreement. *Business Wire*, May 15.

Ransom, Jeanie Franz. 1993. Help is on the phone. *American Baby* 55 (June): 26.

Rauber, Chris. 1994. 21st century vision. *Healthcare Forum*, January–February, 75–78.

Roan, Sheri. 1995. An online medical miasmic: cyberspace bulletin boards offer support and advice on health. *Los Angeles Times*, February 15, A1.

Sasenick, Susan M. 1994. On healthier communities. Supplement to *Healthcare Forum* Vol. 7, No. 3, May–June, 57–72.

Sprenger, Gordon. 1995. Interview with Ken Jennings. Minneapolis, Minn.

Strand, David. 1995. Interview with Sharyn Materna. August 7.

Williams, Thomas R. 1995. Interview with Sharyn Materna, Wendy Kingsbury, and Ken Jennings.

Winslow, Ron. 1995. Unit of Cigna to go outside for its lab tests. *Wall Street Journal*, October 4, B14.

Wolff, Jennifer. 1995. Electronic doctors. *Self* Vol. 17, October, 86.

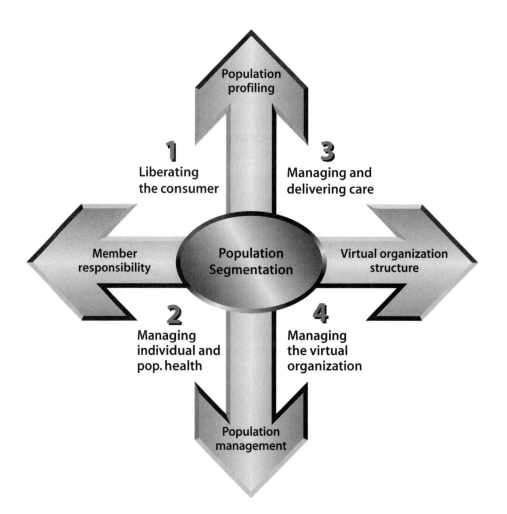

Population
profiling

**1**
Liberating
the consumer

**3**
Managing and
delivering care

Member
responsibility

Population
Segmentation

Virtual organization
structure

**2**
Managing
individual and
pop. health

**4**
Managing
the virtual
organization

Population
management

# PART II

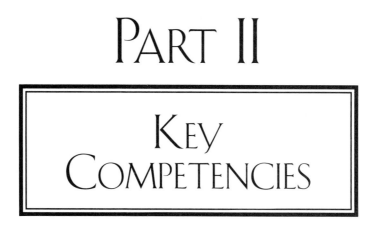

The competencies described in this section are those that are necessary to deliver on the strategies described in Part I. As the industry continues to change, as many new niche players emerge, and as technology enables many different forms of virtual relationships, the competencies that winning health enterprises will need will change dramatically from those that made their past success possible. In this section of the book, we examine four key competencies that health organizations will need to insure their future success:

▼ Liberating the health care consumer

▼ Managing individual and population health

▼ Managing and delivering care

▼ Managing the virtual organization

These four competencies are represented in the figure opposite, which illustrates their collective dependence on population segmentation. By starting with a more sophisticated approach to segmentation, winning health enterprises will be able to develop a supercapability that cuts across all four of the capabilities described in this section. We call this supercapability "Touch and Triage," the ability to build and maintain relationships with individual consumers and guide them through a virtual system for optimal outcomes. This is the real challenge for winning health enterprises of the future.

The significance of these competencies will become even more evident when health organizations realize that what kept them going in the past will not necessarily serve them well in the future. The advantage of location and broad geographic reach will erode as technology continues to make time and distance irrelevant. Providing a broad spectrum of product options will pale in importance compared to the array of choices provided through mass customization. Responsiveness to customer needs will no longer suffice when technology and empowered consumers require organizations to work proactively to anticipate customer needs. Treating member information as proprietary—an advantage in conventional systems—will become a recipe for disaster in the consumer-driven, information-intensive world of the future. And resources such as finances, facilities, providers, and other keys to success in the past will take a backseat to knowledge and the ability to learn and grow.

The capabilities described in this section also cut across almost all functional areas and processes within the winning health enterprise of the future. There is, however, a strong focus on relationships with individual consumers, purchasers, and partners. These relationships are the key to increasing value for the consumer. Additionally, there is a strong emphasis on medical management as medical costs typically account for as much as 90 percent of the overall costs of most health enterprises. Many health care organizations are also beginning to realize that increasing value can be provided only by taking a comprehensive view of what constitutes health care services in the eyes of the consumer—not from the viewpoint of the physician or the health plan.

Figure 11 illustrates why this focus is becoming so important. It depicts three large and overlapping industry change waves. These waves relate to the evolutionary phases touched on briefly in Chapter 1, but we expand our discussion of them here to provide a better context within which to define the four competencies.

As markets progress through various stages of managed care, from loosely managed to tightly managed to a stage beyond tightly managed (which we are beginning to see in markets like those of Northern and Southern California), the rules for success change dramatically. In loosely managed markets, where limited capitation and shared incentives among health plans, providers, and other stakeholders exist, insurers have typically called the shots. As a result, organizations built capabilities that have been focused largely on

*Figure 11* MANAGED CARE EVOLUTION

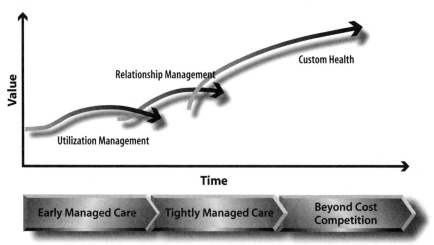

enabling outstanding utilization management to provide low costs to purchasers. Those capabilities were focused on episodes of care dealing with sick patients and were targeted largely at changing physician behavior. That approach has often been suboptimal due to its fragmented nature. It has also frequently frustrated, even enraged, providers. The majority of the organizations we interviewed believe that most of the value, including cost, quality, and service, has already been squeezed out with these approaches, and that continued success will require moving beyond traditional utilization management—and we agree wholeheartedly.

The next wave is what we refer to as relationship and population management. This is more often seen in tightly managed markets, where purchasers are calling the shots by demanding low cost and increased value. The focus on building capabilities is shifting to understanding and responding to the care and service needs of specific, targeted populations. This approach typically targets members with chronic conditions and at high risk and includes programs such as disease and demand management. It is focused on changing both provider and member behavior and takes a more comprehensive delivery system approach across the entire care continuum. While most of the leaders of health enterprises we interviewed have mastered the capabilities necessary within the utilization management wave, far fewer organizations have made significant progress within this area. Those that have, however, are building considerable competitive advantage and are discussed in the following chapters.

We believe there is a stage beyond cost competition, however, which in most markets is just below the horizon. It is the world of custom care, made possible by information technology, active and empowered consumers, the demystification of medicine, and virtual organizations. It is a world beyond the radar screens of many large health services organizations today. A handful of small, entrepreneurial companies, as well as a number of large organizations such as Disney and AT&T that have not historically been players in the health care industry, recognize the potential riches of this new world.

Custom health builds on relationship management by moving to a "segment of one." Doing so means targeting the member individually, focusing on total health needs over time, and operating across a much broader, consumer-defined continuum of health services. Some examples of those services include acupuncture, fitness training, nutritional counseling, and herbal therapy. Custom health focuses on maximizing each member's health potential by understanding not only traditional risk factors but also other psychographic, behavioral, and attitudinal factors.

The evolution of custom health, as you will see in the following chapters, is still at an embryonic stage. Nonetheless, it has the potential to create power shifts within the health care industry similar to the massive changes wrought by the microprocessor in the computer industry, the jet engine in the transportation industry, or quartz technology in the watch industry. In the following chapters we will highlight several early examples of custom health within the current marketplace, and in Chapter 12 (Creating the Future), we will explore some of the long-term opportunities and implications for all health enterprises.

The actual importance of all this, however, revolves around building sustainable capabilities that will allow an organization to excel across all three waves of change simultaneously. This is what Touch and Triage is all about. You will see how it enables building a deep understanding of consumer wants and needs; enables constant sensing of and responding to these ever-changing needs; "triages" members to the products, services, and information they need; and facilitates the "touch" between members and these services.

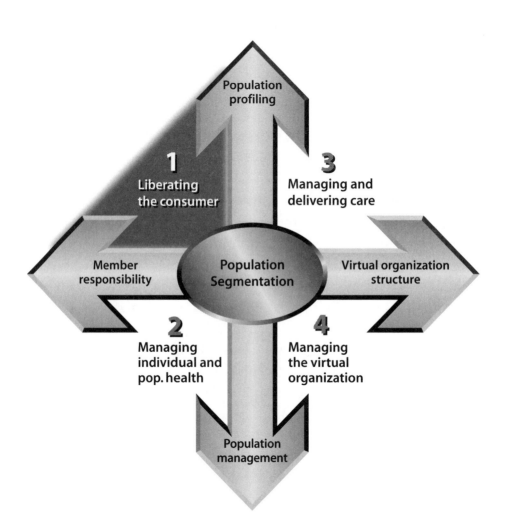

Population
profiling

**1**
Liberating
the consumer

**3**
Managing and
delivering care

Member
responsibility

Population
Segmentation

Virtual organization
structure

**2**
Managing
individual and
pop. health

**4**
Managing
the virtual
organization

Population
management

# 4

## LIBERATING THE CONSUMER

R emember the old Model T? This first car built on
Henry Ford's brainchild, the assembly line, illustrated
that automobiles could be mass produced and
made available in large quantities to thousands of customers.
By utilizing repetition and leveraging economies of scale, automobile manufacturers employed Industrial Age mass-production techniques to make cars that were affordable for the
masses. When it came to consumer preference or choice, however, the popular response was: "You can have any color as long
as it's black."

The auto industry has come a long way since then. Consumers today can walk into a Saturn dealer, sit down at a computer terminal, configure their own options, and specify a
preference for a date of delivery.

Mass-production approaches worked for years in the auto-
motive industry but eventually gave way to a customer-focused,

just-in-time, flexible manufacturing model as consumer demand, technological advances, and stiff competition converged to transform the industry. Winning health enterprises are beginning to realize that similar changes will be necessary in health care to be successful in the future.

Today the health care industry is, for the most part, still operating under the old Industrial Age mass-production model. Many health plans and providers continue to offer benefits packages and care delivery services that are largely one-size-fits-all in nature, despite the fact that we all have different health wants, needs, and preferences.

Consider your own experiences. For years, at annual enrollment time, consumers simply sent in their paperwork to select from a limited set of options such as traditional indemnity coverage, HMO, PPO, or point of service plan. Similarly, many care management and delivery programs targeted at consumers—wellness and prevention, health risk assessment, or even the structure of a routine physician office visit—are also essentially mass produced and distributed, with little differentiaton between individual consumer profiles.

Things are beginning to change. Better and faster information capabilities, a shift toward greater consumer involvement, and heightened competition—between traditional industry players and new market entrants—are forcing health care organizations to understand, engage, and even liberate the consumer. One organization that is converting this approach into greater value and competitive advantage is the Buyers Health Care Action Group (BHCAG) in the Minneapolis/St. Paul metropolitan area. (Buyers 1994)

Since its founding in 1988, the organization has grown into a coalition of 24 self-insured employers including American Express Financial Advisors, Cargill, General Mills, Honeywell, 3M, and 150,000 employees of state and local governments.

BHCAG puts consumers at the center of the health care system and asks physician groups, hospitals, and other care systems to earn these customers' business. Thus, they will sustain customer loyalty with excellent delivery of products and services.

Recently BHCAG contracted with HealthPartners, a non-profit health plan, to develop software that will give customers a user-friendly means of shopping for providers: Employees can check costs, quality of care, customer satisfaction with the 200 clinics in the network, even physicians' credentials, photographs, and personal statements. (Wise 1995)

BHCAG's actions highlight the extensive changes in the health care market and how a winning health enterprise liberates its customers. It is no surprise that consumers want outstanding service, equal to the service they receive from companies in other industries. They yearn for individual treatment, along with a selection of products that closely fit their needs. Ready to participate more actively in decisions about their care, these consumers demand health care organizations recognize that they are discriminating buyers who will shop around for the best doctors, hospitals, services, and procedures and, when properly informed, make intelligent decisions about access and utilization.

To capture this market, health care professionals must clearly understand the needs and preferences of their customers and provide refined systems that guide them to the products and services that suit them best. In short, they must find ways to engage the consumer more effectively across a wide variety of processes to provide the right mix of products and services, configure their delivery networks appropriately, and optimize consumer demand for health care services.

But before the health organization can accomplish this goal, it must first know the consumers in ways that a chart of blood pressure levels or a sonogram of the hepatic artery cannot provide. The first step in this process is segmenting the population.

### Segmenting the Consumer Market

We learn things, in part, by categorizing them. Colleges and universities segment applicants by region, gender, religious affiliation, parental income, SAT scores, and a host of other identifiers. Other industries focus on a single criterion such as customers' credit history or yearly salary. To stay competitive and to keep their customers loyal, health care organizations too must thoroughly know their customers, not just by name but by various market- and member-segmentation categories that help them provide better products and services at lower costs.

Consumer markets have been segmented in other industries by using sets of variables grouped into categories such as demographics, geographics, psychographics, and behavior/attitude. In the past, health care organizations focused largely on demographic and geographic variables to segment their markets and members from a product offering and delivery network architecture perspective. But, as we shall see, these dimensions alone do not always afford the most appropriate features to identify and categorize a population. Many health professionals are beginning to look at consumers' psychographic characteristics and their behaviors and attitudes toward health care: the kinds of benefits and values customers want, how often and for what purposes they use the system, as well as health status indicators such as disease state. This information is then used to configure their programs and delivery networks.

Once segmentation categories are determined, health organizations must seek to engage consumers more proactively to optimize demand for products and services. For example, many health plans and providers today send their members literature on programs designed to help them stop smoking or improve their diets and exercise regimens. Engaging these consumers before they need hospitalization for emphysema or heart bypass surgery will obviously help save both members and health care enterprises vast quantities of money while making consumers more satisfied with their health plans.

From our work with clients in Australia, Singapore, and the United States, we believe that if health care organizations rely solely on the traditional demographic and geographic variables to segment their customers, they will be unable to respond adequately to the rapidly changing market or to optimize the demand for health services for their members. Therefore, in addition to demographics and geographic features, winning health enterprises must incorporate psychographic, behavioral and attitudinal, and health status variables into their approaches to product design, network configuration, and demand optimization programs. This will enable them to design and deliver products and services that keep consumers healthy and loyal.

***Demographic variables:*** Health care organizations are accustomed to segmenting the customer population by demographic factors—age, gender, income, nationality, race, occupation, and the like. In addition, more and more enterprises now use prevalent health status, such as the designation of a specific disease state (diabetes, cancer, or AIDS), to group members and patients. For those groups, care givers then seek to design and administer appropriate services and products, sometimes to the extent of building centers specializing in the treatment of such conditions.

Health care organizations are beginning to combine variables within the category for more precise groupings. They might develop specific programs for women of child-bearing

age who are addicted to drugs, middle-aged men with problems controlling their weight, and children who have cancer.
People suffering from conditions such as sickle-cell anemia,
diabetes, and osteoporosis can benefit from clinical and educational programs based on such segmentation. Obviously,
certain medical problems do not lend themselves to programs, treatments, and services along strictly demographic
lines: While some people may be at a higher risk for contracting HIV, AIDS is not an illness that recognizes age, gender,
ethnic, or sociological boundaries.

Still, demographic segmentation has enormous implications for the future of health care. We are all acutely aware of
the "graying" of America, the projected growth in the number
of people living into their 80s and 90s; for example, the life expectancy for an average 40-year-old is 75 for males and 81 for
females. (Morrison and Schmid 1994; Campion 1993) Given
this eventuality, health care organizations must determine
how to incorporate and combine variables beyond these demographics into specific products and programs to improve
health status and lower costs for this important population
segment.

*Geographic variables:* In addition to using demographic
segmentation, health care organizations have also employed
geographic variables such as region, city, or even neighbor-
hood to help them customize products and programs and
configure their delivery networks. For example, the Henry
Ford Health System has established a network of facilities in
Detroit's inner-city area. These variables are also being used to
help map out population health management plans, such as
immunization, screening, and education programs. Proximity
to certain geographic regions known to have specific health
risks, such as the fact that urban children in Pittsburgh have
increased bronchitis due to secondhand smoke from their

mothers, can alert care givers to anticipate and proactively screen for illnesses like cancer, birth defects, and asthma.

The traditional variables of demographic and geographic segmentation have proved useful to health care organizations in the past. They have, however, begun to encounter a number of natural limits because they have provided few actionable insights about pricing, product features, network delivery architecture, or specific niches. For continued success, health care organizations will need to build on traditional variables and find the right dimension, or more likely the right combination of dimensions, that pertains to its customers by including both psychographic and behavioral/attitudinal variables.

*Psychographic variables:* Less commonly used by health care professionals but no less significant are psychographic features. Does lifestyle influence decisions about health? Is the individual a workaholic? How does he or she learn best? How open is the patient or member to suggestions of changing high-risk behaviors like smoking or consuming alcohol? As evidence mounts linking certain psychographic features with the ability to identify and manage health risk, as well as to influence consumer demand for health services, care givers and insurance providers will look more closely to these segmentation variables to guide their strategies in developing and marketing products and services to purchasers and consumers. A deeper understanding of these factors can also assist health care enterprises design and deliver various disease management, demand management, and other programs to employers, members, patients, and providers.

*Variables related to member's behavior and attitudes toward health care:* Health care organizations know how difficult it is to persuade people to have regular checkups or to participate in other prevention activities such as using seatbelts and helmets or getting pap smears and mammograms. Many, particularly the healthy young, often wait until some significant event such as a pregnancy or catastrophic illness occurs before visiting a doctor. Others want all the care and advice they can get and do not mind waiting or paying for it or, in other cases, having third parties pay for it. These examples illustrate dimensions of both product design and demand optimization.

By using a behavior/attitude segmentation to assist with product design, organizations might discover segments such as a group of price-conscious consumers wanting low monthly premiums that cover the most costly kinds of care but do not cover premium care or optional services. Product features for this group might include low monthly premiums for catastrophic coverage but high copayments and deductibles for optional services.

*Figure 12*  SEGMENTATION VARIABLES

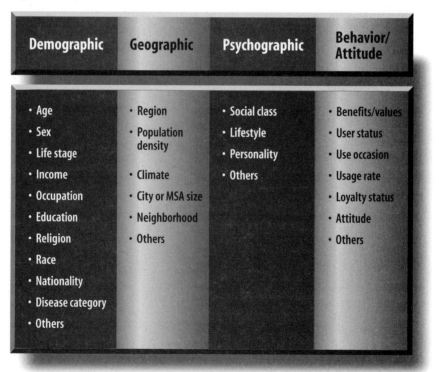

| Demographic | Geographic | Psychographic | Behavior/Attitude |
|---|---|---|---|
| • Age | • Region | • Social class | • Benefits/values |
| • Sex | • Population density | • Lifestyle | • User status |
| • Life stage | | • Personality | • Use occasion |
| • Income | • Climate | • Others | • Usage rate |
| • Occupation | • City or MSA size | | • Loyalty status |
| • Education | • Neighborhood | | • Attitude |
| • Religion | • Others | | • Others |
| • Race | | | |
| • Nationality | | | |
| • Disease category | | | |
| • Others | | | |

Other customers might value choice and relationship above price. They may want to select their providers and determine who has control of their personal health. To appeal to that group, organizations might offer consumers a trusting relationship with physicians and provider teams who routinely spend considerable time learning each consumer's medical history and needs and provide each consumer with a feeling of empathy, security, and respect. (Group Health Association 1995)

This segmentation is not restricted merely to customers' preferences on health care plans. Other factors in this segmentation can become evident as the patient or member becomes more engaged in the health care process. Some members, for example, will reject any suggestion that they quit smoking, even though they may be fully aware of its dangers and have seen graphic pictures of human lungs ravaged by years of smoking. Others, however, will begin to open up to suggestions that they change behaviors; some, indeed, will actively seek to join programs designed to help them give up smoking.

The criteria of actual and perceived health status can also be used to segment the population and develop appropriate responses to its needs. The "worried well" segment, for example, overuses the health care system because of perceived illnesses and problems. Although to the sufferer those vague complaints are all too real, the appropriate response is not unlimited access to a primary care physician but rather education and counseling to eliminate inappropriate utilization and access.

### A Segment of One

As the example of the worried well suggests, segmentation variables do overlap. We believe that it is critical for health organizations to find the right variables or the right combination of variables to provide significant value to customers. Over time, winning health enterprises will need to move from broad population segments, like disease category, to a segment of one. The ideal is to treat each member of an HMO, each patient in a fee-for-service plan, each citizen (whatever his or her insurance or health status may be) as an individual for whom a unique and comprehensive health plan has been designed.

For a large HMO with several million members, this ideal may seem impractical and too costly to implement. But even some of the largest health organizations, as well as demand management vendors like Access Health, are already moving in the direction of customizing a life care plan for each member. As we will see more fully in Chapter 5, several organizations are beginning to build the competency to make such care plans a reality. This type of capability has already been demonstrated in other industries, such as manufacturing and financial services, through an approach called mass customization. Mass customization refers to the ability to prepare on a mass basis individually designed products to meet each customer's requirements. The Saturn example provided earlier is an illustration of this customization, as is the ability of jeans and swimsuit manufacturers to produce custom-fitted apparel.

No health care enterprise has yet developed an end-all, superior formula for comprehensively segmenting health care consumers, and given the complexity of health issues, the most effective segmentation will vary from organization to organization. Ultimately, however, leaders of the winning health care enterprise have to ask, "What services and products are we going to offer our health care customers? And how can we engage them more proactively in their own health to optimize demand for these services?"

### Segmentation in Practice

Andersen Consulting recently worked with a large health provider whose use of segmentation provides important insights into how products can be tailored for members. Recognizing that members are very different in their attitudes toward health care, this enterprise is developing a set of four options to appeal to young and old. Rather than forcing all members to pay the same monthly charges for the same health care coverage and services, the organization will offer several plans that give them a variety of options. One of these plans will cater to a group that is highly price sensitive and willing to forgo many choice and service options. This product may appeal most to relatively young, healthy members who do not anticipate needing many medical services and are therefore less concerned about choice.

This organization will also provide plans that offer members abundant choice of primary care physicians and specialists. Care givers' credentials as well as personal interests and traits may be made available to plan members who would be liberated to make their choices accordingly. A 35-year-old woman with a family history of uterine cancer, for instance, might choose a gynecologist who combines her specialty training with work in oncology.

Still a third set of products envisioned by this organization revolves around the issue of relationship. This member segment places a high priority on the quality of the relationship with its plan and providers and the role that these strong relationships play in avoiding medical risk.

Recognizing that there is a fourth category of customers, namely those who want it all, the organization seeks to provide another option that attempts to balance all three of the value points outlined here, without placing undue emphasis on any one.

Another innovator in this arena is Aetna. Indeed, Aetna's leaders have taken the next step in effectively utilizing market segmentation by asking the question that all plan providers need to ask: "Once members are enrolled, how can we best engage them in care management, delivery, and service processes?" After surveying members on their experiences and preferences for health care coverage, Aetna segmented customers around a number of variables, including general member characteristics and demographics, as well as satisfaction and loyalty levers. This segmentation process resulted in five broad population segments.

Twenty-two percent of the population is defined as informed decision makers: They take an active interest in health matters and show an ability to manage their own health care. Twenty-three percent of the population is most concerned about the right to select physicians to whom they are loyal and with whom they have developed trust and caring. Twenty-seven percent of the population may be confused and frustrated with the health care marketplace. What these people demand is efficient, straightforward service, without the medical jargon or the runaround that poisons so many relationships between care givers and their clients. Eighteen percent of the population runs essentially on autopilot: They expect and respond well to efficient services and a broad choice of products.

The remaining 10 percent of the population appears apathetic, uninterested, and uninvolved with health care issues. No amount of clever advertising or outreach connects with this segment, who are low utilizers and do not appear to have any health concerns. Typically the health care organization must wait for a health event to trigger these individuals' interaction with the system.

Aetna's innovative approach illustrates how a large managed care organization can analyze the values its customers have toward health care and use that analysis to develop appropriate products, services, and responses. It seeks to give customers what they want, at the same time anticipating what they need to keep them healthy.

Another segmentation approach gaining momentum across markets is that offered by the health risk and disease management provider Healthtrac. Healthtrac's program has been purchased by a number of health care organizations, which use it to identify potential high-risk members and group them into population segments such as arthritis, back pain, a history of cigarette smoking, diabetes, high blood pressure, lung disease, and health problems due to pregnancy. Once these high-risk members are identified, Healthtrac provides ways to manage them along specific disease paths. Thus Healthtrac offers a health promotion and disease prevention product, available through employer health plans, that segments subscribers into many different groups according to customer questionnaires. All Healthtrac subscribers complete a detailed questionnaire about their health complaints, medical and family histories, and lifestyles. Healthtrac then sends each subscriber recommendations about care, healthy behaviors, lifestyle changes, and self-management.

To each group, Healthtrac mails a sequence of questionnaires at three- to six-month intervals. Based on consumers' answers, the program then sends the high-risk subscribers various books, audiotapes, and videos. Utilizing innovative technology, nurses keep tabs on subscribers by phone or occasionally intervene with counseling, medication, behavior therapy, and other follow-up as needed. (Blackwood 1992; Brooks 1993)

The use of Healthtrac reduces the number of doctor visits, hospital stays, and sick days. Even Healthtrac's standard program for healthy subscribers saved more than twice its cost. As Healthtrac has shown repeatedly in randomized controlled trials, the segmenting of consumers yields a double win: keeping people healthier and reducing costs for the organization.

### Engaging Consumers to Optimize Demand

As illustrated above, part of Healthtrac's approach to managing care is the proactive engagement of the consumer. Recent studies demonstrate the importance of this engagement in optimizing consumer demand. As little as 12 percent of all variation and utilization of medical services (for example, visits to physicians and hospitals) can be attributed to actual morbidity. The other 88 percent results from either personal preferences, perceived need, nonhealth motives, or unexplained factors (see Figure 13). (Vickery and Lynch 1996) Moreover, Caresoft, Inc., of San Jose, California, estimates that up to 70 percent of illnesses are preventable. (Lazarus 1995: 54–59) Demand optimization aims to eliminate those drivers of unnecessary care and to encourage consumers to use health care services as medical conditions merit.

**Figure 13** A LESSON IN OPPORTUNITY

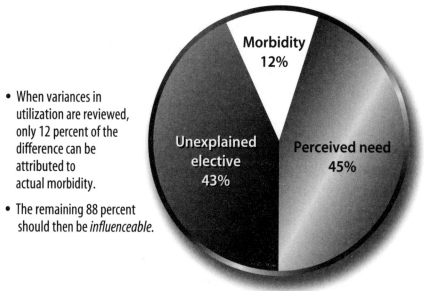

• When variances in utilization are reviewed, only 12 percent of the difference can be attributed to actual morbidity.

• The remaining 88 percent should then be *influenceable*.

Morbidity 12%

Unexplained elective 43%

Perceived need 45%

*Modified from Healthier Communities Direct (Agfa Division, Bayer Corporation) "New Disease Management"; by Don Vickery (Health Decisions International, LLC)*

There are two principal ways to attack the drivers of unnecessary care: create incentives to change consumer behavior and disseminate information at the right time to the right person to influence consumers' decisions. As organizations find the correct combinations to use in segmenting their populations, they can better tailor educational materials to encourage appropriate care levels. Wellness handbooks, decision-making software, and online support groups can help many people care for themselves, reducing the overall, long-term demand for professional care. The idea is to alter people's tendency to visit the doctor or hospital into a tendency to visit the library or consult the expert system on their PC.

Organizations can also optimize demand by virtualizing services through the use of information technology to link consumers to care givers who specialize in home monitoring services or telemedicine. They can develop more precise on-line care paths to coordinate preventive, primary, and acute care and avoid waste and duplication of care and services. In addition, they can employ nurses in sophisticated phone counseling services that divert consumers from expensive facilities and practitioners. One study in Colorado showed that in fielding 400,000 calls, a nurse triage call center could resolve 60 percent of calls over the phone. Nurses directed 25 percent of the callers to a physician's office the next day, and only 15 percent required immediate attention in an emergency room. (Lazarus 1995) Through more intensive use of information to connect directly to consumers, organizations can shrink the demand for care and more effectively deploy scarce resources across the system.

Kaiser Permanente, for example, is considering a set of ten services under the name Kaiser Permanente Direct (KP Direct). Although it is still in the planning stages, Kaiser Permanente Direct will target consumers with three products: care path planning, symptom evaluation, and disease management. Using the care path planning product, consumers will be able to customize all prevention and lifestyle decisions to their specific needs, taking into account age, gender, occupation, known diseases, and other personal factors. Care path planning will give consumers targeted educational materials, appointment reminders, care guidelines, and a way to communicate with their care givers at Kaiser Permanente.

KP Direct will provide a symptom evaluation tool to help consumers narrow the possible causes of an illness simply by answering a series of questions about early symptoms and conditions. Eventually customers will complete such questionnaires on home computers rather than at the doctor's office or in an emergency room. According to Chris Dinnin of Andersen Consulting, a member of the core planning team for this project, one of the objectives is to reduce the number of unnecessary visits to primary care physicians and better prepare the patient and provider for their in-person encounter. Some surveys put unnecessary visitation as high as 60 percent. (Dinnin 1995)

Once the list of causes has been reduced, the program will evaluate the relative merits of various levels of care, self-care, a visit to an outpatient clinic, or admission through an emergency room. Rather than relying primarily on members' medical histories to make diagnoses, Kaiser Permanente Direct will guide members through the questionnaire and treatment options before recommending a course of care.

Using Kaiser Permanente Direct's disease management product, consumers will receive information on specific diseases, along with self-help tools for monitoring, evaluating, and treating them. The disease management offering will also dispense advice on lifestyle and social issues, remind consumers about appointments, and include a tracking system for treatment. ("Kaiser Permanente Direct Initiative" 1995)

One of the virtues of Kaiser Permanente Direct and similar programs is that customers take a greater sense of responsibility for their health and participate in the cure of an illness or management of their health. They know that they can no longer afford to sit back and passively receive treatments.

Much as Kaiser Permanente has developed these new products, Aetna Health Plans, with its custom health offering, is pursuing its version of consumer empowerment. Both organizations are planning to provide virtual products through information services that put the consumer and the organization in touch through telecommunications, rather than through costly and far more inconvenient office and clinic visits. Kaiser Permanente Direct and custom health will offer exactly what consumers want: convenience, better health, more control and better access, informed decision making, and a sense of ownership of their own care. Taking their cue from organizations like Kaiser Permanente and Aetna, health care enterprises will develop similar products to meet customers' demands.

As Robert A. Lauer, Andersen Consulting's managing partner for Change Management in the Americas, observes, it is no longer enough for a health care organization to treat only pain and illness: "When you are in the business of preventive medicine, then you have to understand people's lifestyles, habits, living patterns, demographics, and buying practices. That's what segmentation is all about." (Lauer 1996)

Liberating the consumer, therefore, is in large part a function of educating the consumer. If they are to hold the reins on excessive spending, health care organizations will have to provide that education, teaching people how to make smart use of the health care system's resources and personnel. As we saw in Chapter 3, the tremendous growth in telephone and Internet information services has the potential to reduce the number and frequency of unnecessary medical visits. In addition, wellness and prevention programs will incorporate educational materials to help people make better use of the system. Given the degree of interest that people now take in their own health, we can be encouraged to envision a future in which health care professionals focus on guiding consumers to appropriate information and access options, as well as treating chronic and acute diseases, catastrophic illnesses, and true medical emergencies.

### Creating the Network Architecture

How quickly and effectively the health organization responds to customers' needs and optimizes demand will be a function largely of the efficiency and structure of providers who make up the service delivery network. In liberating their consumers, winning health enterprises must discover new ways to engage them in helping to manage their own health and in making better use of the health care system. They must also think more broadly about what constitutes a comprehensive network architecture.

Figure 14, for example, illustrates a potential configuration for a group model HMO with one million covered lives. In this possible future, members have been segmented into a set of populations managed by a combination of individual providers and teams. The delivery network includes service and delivery channels such as call centers, online care, and video clinics to optimize its response to member demand. Nontraditional services such as acupuncture and health clubs are included for members who value these services. In such a network, and with the innovations described in Chapters 5–7, the costs of providing care and service are likely to be much lower than those of today's best-performing groups.

This type of future configuration will require significant

*Figure 14* AN ADVANCED GROUP PRACTICE MODEL

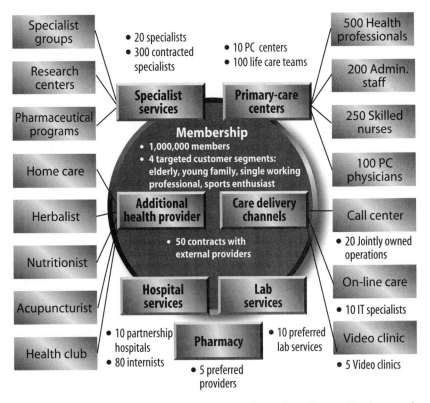

innovations in people, process, and technology. Perhaps the most significant of these potential innovations will be the portable medical record, which health care professionals will be able to access anywhere in the world whenever they need it. Whether one is seeing a primary care physician or specialist in his/her office, undergoing surgery at a regional center of excellence, or receiving advice from the call center nurse, each of the virtual team members will have access to the most up-to-date, accurate, and relevant information. Additionally, we will eventually have the peace of mind that comes with knowing that, should something go wrong, a complete record of all illnesses, treatments, wellness programs, and health care concerns will be available online.

An early example of this capability is provided by Access HealthNet, which currently provides management and communications systems to physicians, hospitals, laboratories, and other health care organizations that make up the Alameda Alliance for Health in Oakland, California. With connections to other areas of the country, Access HealthNet will allow physicians in, say, Virginia to confer with colleagues in California through Remote ACCESS; similar linkage is possible between laboratories and community networks. According to Stephen Levy, CEO of Access HealthNet, "The market for remote medical communication products is currently $800 million annually and is expanding at 35 percent per year. The domestic market . . . includes approximately 7,500 clinical laboratories and in excess of 6,500 hospitals."(Levy 1995; see also "Access HealthNet" 1995)

Also moving rapidly toward this virtual future of health care, Access Health, Inc., of Rancho Cordova, California, offers an excellent example of an organization that incorporates up-to-date processes to improve service delivery to its customers. This innovative organization is developing ways to match its ten million members (including all employees and retirees of General Motors Corporation, as well as their dependents) to various resources across its virtual health care system. Through online connections and telephone access, care givers speak to eligible members about medical problems, offering advice and referral, screening calls that require immediate attention, and enabling members to manage their own health. For a small monthly fee, individual subscribers, even if they move or change health plans, can access the Personal Health Advisor, a telephone triage service staffed by trained medical personnel.

The results of Access Health's service have been outstanding: The organization has realized cost savings up to 28 percent. (Group Health Association 1995) In its pilot program offered to 125,000 members in western Pennsylvania, the research library and staff of online nurses received 4,500 calls, fewer than 300 of which concerned medical emergencies. Seventy-five percent of those calls were requests for medical information. (Barnet 1995)

Such uses of information technology only begin to suggest the many possibilities for more effectively engaging the consumer and optimizing demand. Information technology can be applied to engage consumers and optimize demand at four levels: facilitation, demystification, participation, and disintermediation. As a *facilitator*, information technology gives consumers the ability to interact with their health providers at any time. For example, the organization might offer online query systems and phone systems manned by nurses equipped with computers that give consumers fast and convenient access to information and counsel.

Dr. Vincent Riccardi, an advocate for American Medical Consumers, advises consumers to learn to speak some of the language of the medical profession. Nothing gets quicker attention than a layperson talking to the staff at the nursing facility "about jargon items such as MDS [minimal data set] and the RAP [resident action plan]." (Riccardi 1996) Mastery of the lingo allows consumers to take greater control over their health care. By *demystifying* the profession's jargon, information technology can help consumers discover facts, statistics, and arguments to understand complex medical issues.

Thanks to the wonders of modern technology, consumers today have a greater sense of *participation* in their own care. They can readily access medical knowledge and become better informed about their conditions. When it comes time to work with their care givers, they can make well-informed decisions. Such participation will improve outcomes, ultimately reduce costs, and increase the consumer's satisfaction with care.

*Disintermediation* is the last level of technology-enabled interaction and refers to the removal of all barriers: the non-value-adding people and processes that do not directly facilitate the consumers' ability to receive needed medical service, information, or treatment. For certain groups of health savvy consumers and people with selected medical needs, this may even mean eliminating the need for interaction with a provider. In a fully disintermediated situation, consumers will have the necessary information to diagnose and even treat themselves. Many examples of this disintermediation already exist, such as diabetics who maintain tighter control of their own glucose levels or cancer patients who do their own research and design their own treatment plans.

We can also see the early effects of those technologies in the explosion of new programs of online services. For about $40, subscribers to America Online and other services can purchase a CD-ROM produced by the American Medical Association that promises to help them find answers to many of their health care questions. Simply by typing in the keyword "health," for example, America Online members can gain access to the Better Health and Medical Forum, receive the latest information on health problems and treatments, learn about alternative medicines, and gain access to MEDLINE, a huge database of medical information. ("America Online" 1995)

The achievements of Access HealthNet suggest additional approaches that winning health care enterprises will use to supplement the traditional face-to-face encounter between physician and patient. While these face-to-face encounters will not completely disappear in the future health care world, they may not be the primary mode for diagnosing illnesses, prescribing treatments, or establishing relationships with consumers. Virtual relationships provided through telephone hotlines and referral services, computer-accessible databases, multimedia educational software, interactive television, and interactive health care kiosks are just a few of the developments that establish consumers' long-term partnership with their health care organizations.

The wide communications capabilities that enterprises such as Access HealthNet and others provide will also help to break down traditional barriers between health care administrators and care givers. In the past, consumers worked with administrative personnel to enroll in a health plan or acquire indemnity insurance. Unless they came down with the flu, broke a leg, or suffered a heart attack, consumers remained invisible to care givers in the organization. Only then would their records cross from administration to care delivery. With the new interactive media and technology, however, customer service processes can render the member's enrollment and receipt of health care a seamless operation.

The merging of databases and the integration of administrative and clinical processes will unleash scores of possibilities for new services, one of the most important of which is the life care plan. A concept that began as not much more than a computerized plan for long-term individual care, the life care plan will grow much more sophisticated. Rendered feasible by integrated software systems, each care path could ultimately include a consumer profile, a thin slice of clinical and administrative information, and links to all relevant clinical and administrative systems, including billing, claims, care guidelines, and medical outcomes systems.

As we will see in the next chapter, the life care plan and life care teams are crucial components in the competency of managing the health of individuals and entire populations.

As the health care industry works through this period of chaos, long-term relationships between consumers and care providers will grow, requiring more frequent contact. The paradox, however, is that to keep costs down, the health organization must try to minimize contact. Winning enterprises will devise ways to resolve that paradox, primarily by creating high-touch, low-cost information and triage services. As both Access Health and Access HealthNet show, there is much to gain from liberating the consumer through technologies that create virtual relationships with care givers.

Organizations must develop more highly refined systems to guide consumers to the services that suit them best, whether they are acutely ill, chronically ill, prone to illness, or just looking for reassurance and wellness counseling. As new capabilities emerge, health care organizations will encourage consumers to take far more responsibility for their own care. At the same time, consumers will force action by health care organizations. The new focus on the consumer implies change for the customers of health care, but it implies far more change for health care organizations, which face the challenges of simultaneously revamping technology, pro-cesses, people, skills, and even organizational culture. As the organization surveys its key competencies, it must seek ways to liberate consumers by engaging them in the complex pro-cesses of health care management and delivery.

# REFERENCES

Access HealthNet announces agreement with Unilab. 1995. PRNewswire, October 3.

America Online announces the launch of new online health area. 1995. Individual, Inc., October 13.

Barnet, Alice Ault. 1995. Is knowledge really power for patient? *Business & Health* 13 (May): 29.

Blackwood, Francy. 1992. Healthy business: employee wellness programs. *California Business*, December, 17.

Brooks, Nancy Rivera. 1993. Wellness's weakening pulse: companies rethink programs in effort to trim health costs. *Los Angeles Times*, February 25, D1.

Buyers (Business) Health Care Action Group. 1994. Annual report.

Campion, Edward W. 1993. Why unconventional medicine? *New England Journal of Medicine*, January 28, 282–83.

Dinnin, Chris. 1995. Interview with Erik Hansen. December 13.

Group Health Association of America. 1995. A Future for Healthcare. Andersen Consulting. Information Management Conference and Exposition. November 29. Unpublished manuscript.

Kaiser Permanente Direct Initiative: advisory group work session (San Francisco, Calif.). 1995. Unpublished report. Andersen Consulting. November 1.

Lauer, Robert A. 1996. Interview with Ken Jennings.

Lazarus, Ian R. 1995. Medical call centers. *Managed Healthcare*, October, Vol. 5, No. 10, 54–59.

Levy, Stephen. 1995. Access HealthNet letter to stockholders. October 18. (PRNewswire)

Morrison, Ian, and Greg Schmid. 1994. *Future tense: the business realities of the next ten years.* New York: William Morrow and Company.

Riccardi, Vincent. 1996. Interview with Kurt Miller and Susan Vanderpool.

Vickery, M.D., Donald M., and Wendy Lynch, Ph.D. 1996. Demand management: enabling patients to use medical care appropriately. *Healthcare Forum*, January–February.

Wise, Dan. 1995. Direct contracting comes to the HMO heartland. *Business & Health*, September, 53–54.

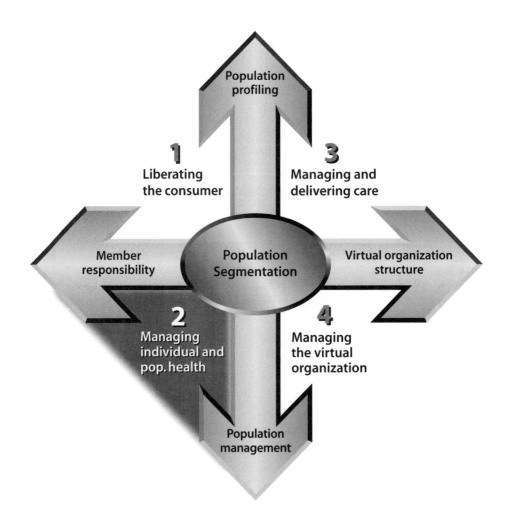

Population
profiling

**1**
Liberating
the consumer

**3**
Managing and
delivering care

Member
responsibility

Population
Segmentation

Virtual organization
structure

**2**
Managing
individual and
pop. health

**4**
Managing
the virtual
organization

Population
management

# 5

## MANAGING INDIVIDUAL AND POPULATION HEALTH

When United HealthCare and MetraHealth announced in June 1995 that they would merge, top executives charged a planning group with choosing the combined firm's top ten priorities. The planning group came back with a list of ten initiatives aimed at solving several problems related to the merger, such as how to coordinate existing and new computer systems. To the executives' disappointment, not one of the ten pressed the company to pursue emerging opportunities in health care. (Burke 1995)

Given the planning group's short-term focus, top executives wouldn't bless the list. "They were saying their capacity for assimilation of change was at zero tolerance," says Terry Burke, then MetraHealth's senior executive vice president. "We cannot as an organization just deal with temporary operating problems. There has to be some capacity for additional change."

Top executives asked the committee to rework the list and include two of management's favored initiatives: chronic disease management, which aims to help diabetics, asthmatics, hypertensives, and others to stay healthy; and virtual health, a service for coordinating every customer's care by assigning a specific doctor-nurse team to tend to the needs of each patient 24 hours a day, seven days a week.

The two favored choices by United HealthCare executives, who consummated their merger on October 2, 1995, underscored the growing belief in the demand side of health care—providing education, preventive care, and other services in advance of sickness that debilitates the consumer.

United HealthCare executives are putting top priority on developing the second of the four key competencies that winning health care organizations in the future must master, what we call managing individual and population health: providing products and services to promote wellness, prevent illness, identify diseases early, and proactively manage chronic illnesses for individuals and groups. It includes an assessment of health risks, for the individual and the community, as well as ways to manage health through care planning, wellness programs, education, and monitoring of members' health status. What services and products can the organization provide to keep customers healthy?

Effectively managing this side of the equation will require health services organizations to develop more advanced and targeted capabilities in two areas: prevention and disease management. Preventive strategies, which are intended to address avoidable disease states, must be developed and integrated into a consumer-focused approach. Researchers have estimated that as much as 80 percent of health care costs are the result of preventable disease states. Traditional wellness initiatives, however, have not resulted in impact anywhere near this magnitude. To achieve these types of benefits, the information obtained during the population segmentation process described in Chapter 4 must be combined and integrated with an individually customized and tailored approach for each consumer.

Disease-management strategies, which include defined protocols, integrated care management teams, and innovative access points, are the second areas of focus. Many health service organizations have developed a variety of programs in this area. A Southwest staff model HMO, for example, has defined 18 separate disease-management initiatives, including asthma/COPD, chest pain, pneumonia, and low back pain. These programs will provide the protocols and tools to enable virtual care teams to leverage physician extenders and call centers to aggressively manage down the costs of these diseases while improving quality of care and customer satisfaction. Innovative partnerships between health plans and academic centers such as Tufts in Boston and Cedars-Sinai in Los Angeles are leveraging clinical information to create improved disease-management tools, which will further enable health plans to understand and implement best practices across various disease states.

From our vantage point, these innovative approaches to prevention and disease management are necessary but not sufficient to deliver world-class capability in the area of managing personal and population health. As you will see throughout the remainder of this chapter, we believe excelling at this competency will require health service organizations to move beyond these mass market prevention and disease-management approaches to an individualized and customized approach to maximizing consumers' health potential.

In this chapter we examine the key elements of this competency, which we believe the winning health enterprise will require to manage care for individuals and populations: health risk appraisals and member health planning, the life care plan, the life care team, and the proactive management of disease and health risks.

## Assessing Health Risks

The first step in managing health is assessing and understanding health risks at both the individual consumer and population levels. When a health care organization begins cataloging each consumer's current and likely health problems, it builds a foundation of information for preventive care, as well as for proactive management of chronic conditions. At the same time, health care organizations can encourage consumers to commit themselves to taking greater responsibility for their own health, thereby fostering the earliest possible care for latent health problems.

Many health organizations have developed plans for utilizing a variety of health assessment tools and vehicles for new member wellness assessment. Indeed, virtually every large health plan in California now does its own assessment or contracts with others to do it for them. In addition, Pac Bell and other employers in various regions of the country are taking the same initiative to improve the overall health and corresponding productivity of their employees. They collect and analyze specific data on members' or employees' states of health and identify potential health risks.

These organizations are using a variety of approaches to collect this information. Typically, some type of health risk assessment tool is utilized. In the first step of the assessment process, the organization captures a variety of data regarding the individual and his or her health issues. The data varies considerably from organization to organization, depending on the assessment tool being used, as well as the specific objectives the health appraisal process seeks to fulfill. The types of information commonly collected include some degree of medical/health history, demographic and environmental data (age, sex, location, work hazards, etc.), lifestyle and behavioral data (diet, smoking, alcohol use, exercise, etc.), and perceived current health status. Additional data, such as psychographic factors (preferences, social network, etc.) and other unique elements, may also be collected, depending on the specific objectives and assessment tool being used.

One of the issues these organizations need to confront is the proliferation of health risk assessment tools. There are dozens of different tools being marketed today, each with its own emphasis, objectives, and capabilities. Determining how these tools fit into the overall health management process is an important step toward determining which tools and approaches to use. For example, Kaiser Permanente's Northern California Region is running a pilot program with two of its member populations: members over the age of 65 and women between 18 and 44. This program is intended to explore the viability of developing life care paths for KPNCR enrollees. They are using the Dartmouth Coop health risk assessment tool for the 65-plus group to collect functional status information. A customized addendum also obtains diagnosis, medication, and family history information. For the women's program, Kaiser Permanente is using an assessment tool from Eris Survey Systems that obtains lifestyle, modifiable behavior, and screening history information. These survey results and health goals are then used to drive the development of a life care path, which is individually customized for each member.

With this data, the organization can develop a care path for each member that is enrolled in the pilot program. It thus creates a holistic view of consumers and of their needs, from suggested changes in lifestyle to regimens of preventive care such as routine mammograms, blood pressure screenings, and immunizations.

A small number of leading-edge organizations are looking for ways to fold the health assessment and analysis activities into the actual enrollment process. For most members, the enrollment process begins in the workplace. Those organizations envision giving members the option to transfer demographic and family information directly from their personnel files into the health care organization's enrollment database. Because of the impact they can have on overall employee and member health, the organizations are investigating these options despite the inevitable concerns about confidentiality. Members may even be able to enroll from a variety of locations with the aid of interactive television, automated telephones, and home computers.

The enrollment process can then become the launching pad for a new set of valuable preventive and wellness services, and automated enrollment systems would incorporate many of the traditional health risk appraisal questions into the enrollment process, such as "How would you rate your current health?" and "Are there any health problems that concern you?" The enrollee, perhaps noting high blood pressure as a problem and listing current medications, might find the system asking, "What kinds of stress do you experience? What exercise do you engage in most frequently? Do you have a history of high blood pressure in your family?"

Occupational Health Strategies and other firms have developed tools that market self-administered surveys to members of managed care organizations and insurance plan subscribers. These questionnaires elicit information about health history and lifestyle behaviors. When the results are tabulated, members learn about their personal risk for disease as well as steps they can take to reduce it. Occupational Health pioneered 30-year risk projections, which help people understand what they must do to improve their health over the long term. ("Greenstone Healthcare" 1995)

The health assessment also provides a chance for the health care organization to judge each consumer's readiness for change. Lifestyle changes—smoking, eating, drinking, exercise—can have an enormous impact on health. Often, though, the organization must not only identify unhealthy behaviors but also determine the most effective means to encourage the consumer to change.

### The Life Care Plan

We believe the essence of health management and planning will be the life care plan, an ever-changing document that seeks to help members maximize their health potential by focusing on prevention, wellness, and the proactive management of chronic conditions. Life care plans are revolutionary in that they represent the convergence and integration of three powerful forces for change within the health care industry: (1) the redefinition of the relationship between health plan and member from an acute, episode-driven focus to a partnership based on member wellness over time; (2) the use of technology to enable individualization of service while coordinating care across the continuum; and (3) the increased focus on health outcomes as a means to evaluate and improve the effectiveness and efficiency of care delivery processes and systems.

Kaiser Permanente's Northern California Region has been a leader in exploring the development of life care plans for its members. According to Andrea Share, manager for Kaiser Permanente's Life Care Path project, pilot programs were established for the two populations mentioned earlier: members over 65 years of age and women between 18 and 44. (Share 1996) Established in February and March of 1996, respectively, these pilot programs have been initially well received by members and providers and are being used to evaluate the potential benefits and feasibility of rollout to other member segments.

Life care plans can be used by providers, health plan staff, members, and other stakeholders to manage the relationship between the member and his or her health plan and care delivery system over time. In terms of impact, life care plans, taken within the context of personal and population health management, can be a powerful tool that provides substantive benefits to members, providers, and other stakeholders. Members benefit from life care plans as a simple and explicit way to appreciate the big picture of their health and the opportunities they now have to partner with their providers and health plan and influence their quality of life over time. Life care plans can also enhance members' perception of personalized service by providing a predictable, planned schedule of activities for wellness and chronic disease management.

Within KPNCR's pilot programs the life care paths are generated from analysis and output of the health risk assessment surveys. This output is downloaded into a life care path software engine, which uses predefined guidelines and algorithms to specify a set of customized interventions focused on prevention, wellness, and proactive management of any chronic conditions. The life care path engine generates two versions of these member-specific life care paths: a member copy and a provider copy. The member copy is either sent to the member and discussed over the phone or reviewed during a prescheduled visit. This member copy provides a basic set of demographic data, an overall summary of key health risks, and a recommended set of activities, which are fundamental to the life care path. It includes three sections: first, the information and activities that the member can employ on his or her own concerning diet, exercise, selected clinical data collection such as glucose levels for diabetics, etc.; second, the things that the member can do with support from his or her provider team (preventive exams such as PAPs, mammograms, etc.); and third, a listing of all recommended activities in the form of an actual monthly and yearly calendar. This calendar is based on a combination of the guidelines and protocols mentioned previously, as well as actual member-specific clinical information. For example, within the women's program this calendar takes into account the date of the member's last PAP and mammogram when scheduling look-ahead activities. The member copy of the life care path also includes a list of reference materials such as the "Healthwise Handbook," along with other KPNCR support resources and contact information.

The provider copy is a one-page summary placed in the member's chart. This summary is used by providers to step into interactions with the patient quickly and easily and to prompt them to ask members how they are progressing with their recommended activities, remind members of upcoming activities, and reinforce suggested behavior changes.

The life care plans become the backbone of managing a member's health and, as we shall see in the next chapter, the backbone of coordinating care delivery. It is essentially a collection of both ongoing and episodic care plans, for prevention, wellness, intervention, and treatment, all woven together into a highly individualized fabric. The life care plan both helps members enhance their health and aids providers in coordinating health services seamlessly across a continuum of providers.

Note that the life care plan is a frequently changing document, reflecting the member's evolving health status and the care he or she receives. With its thoroughness, it becomes far more vital to health care than today's version of the patient chart. High-risk members can be quickly identified and either channeled into case management programs or proactively linked into other programs focused on reducing these risk factors, such as disease management. When the member phones the nurse advice line to report pain or other symptoms, a nurse can look directly into the care plan, view the patient's history, and make an informed decision about how to proceed. In the past, nurses and doctors simply did not have the information at hand to judge the background health of the patient or the relationship to the current complaint. Nor did they have the predetermined suggestions of the member-specific life care plan to provide the appropriate context and to help guide them in making diagnoses and prescribing interventions.

Many organizations will expand the enrollment and life care planning processes in a variety of directions to build a stronger competency in managing individual and population health. For one thing, the life care plan can incorporate an immense number of details about each consumer, details on which physicians and other care givers can call whenever needed: benefits information; preferred doctors, locations, and pharmacies; and advance care directives (such as living wills, durable powers of attorney, and do-not-resuscitate orders). In addition, the care plans can enable the organization to create a variety of new services to build additional value for the consumer. These plans, customized for each member, will specify concrete goals, education, services, and compliance tracking. The member will then consult the plan as needed to fine-tune his or her health care program.

A particularly important service is tracking the member's compliance. In the past, poor health management frequently resulted from a member's inability or unwillingness to take advantage of either primary or secondary preventive health services. The life care plan specifically calls for care givers to encourage healthy lifestyles and preventive care, even when it means frequent reminders to the patient. In this way, the care plan becomes a working document for case management and communication of health information to both the member and the team of doctors, nurses, and other care givers.

Yet another service that can spring from the life care plan is the health status report. Personalized reports can give consumers direct feedback on their success in managing their health. Such report cards can summarize the tests and procedures performed since the last report; list the classes attended; identify any active wellness, preventive, or chronic care plans; and assess current and future health risks. Members can use this report to keep tabs on their own progress, while physicians use the report to help counsel members on better managing their health.

For a vertically integrated health care organization like Kaiser Permanente Northern California Region, the life care plan requires careful management to bring people and technology together in creative and innovative ways. The care plan must collect and process a tremendous quantity of information about members' health risks, histories, habits, and hopes. This is tricky enough in staff and group model HMOs. It is even more complicated with virtual organizations, which, as we shall see in Chapter 7, must rely on information that is shared across organizational walls.

In the past, health care organizations used technology to improve the efficiency of the laboratory, the radiology department, and other administrative and support services. But the single life care tool integrates the work of all departments and professional staff. Ultimately, it will access and link enrollment data, health assessment rules, scheduling rules, noncompliance rules, survey data, selected clinical data, claim events, case management plans, wellness/preventive/chronic care protocols, and care paths. With so much data tied together and immediately available, care professionals will have a more complete view of their customers than in the past. As a result of this personalized care, rather than the impersonal treatment they may associate with the health care industry, customers are not only more likely to stay healthy, but at KPNCR the belief is that they will also remain more loyal to their health plan and care team.

## The Life Care Team

Life care plans, in short, document and facilitate nearly all of the subprocesses that go into building the competency of managing individual and population health. Successful health care enterprises of the future will place increasing reliance on them to help their members maximize their health potential and build the level of value that consumers expect.

Building this competency will also require significant changes in care giver roles, responsibilities, and relationships. Primary care physicians, for example, will have to adapt to new roles as the industry strengthens its competency in managing individual and population health. To date, primary care physicians have increasingly been cast in the role of gatekeepers, directing to other physicians and higher-cost sources of care only those cases that genuinely demand a specialist. Yet physicians and other providers, such as nurse practitioners, physician assistants, and even medical assistants, will begin to take on far more preventive care work, regularly and routinely seeing patients to counsel them on the practices of healthy living and screening them to catch the onset of any ailments before they become debilitating, costly, and hard to treat.

Care givers will find that effectively managing health demands that they join in care teams to coordinate and deliver comprehensive health services across the entire continuum. Because of the varying needs of each consumer, the teams will be ad hoc and virtual, assembling as needed to match the health profile of each consumer. The practitioners on these teams will have more skills and be more mobile to accommodate consumers' demands.

The composition of each care team will vary and change as the consumer wants and needs change. As illustrated in Figure 15, these care teams will be tailored to the individual needs of the member. An elderly person, for example, might choose a care team composed of a geriatrist, nursing home personnel, a specialty skilled nurse, a nutritionist, a pharmacist, and a dentist. Depending on the consumers' needs, as they develop, it would be possible to add a physical therapist, a speech pathologist, an exercise coach, or a social worker.

### Population Health Management and Outcomes

The third prime element in health management is managing the health of populations and communities. Although health care will continue to include many individually focused relationships between care givers and consumers, health care organizations planning to maximize the collective health of their members must focus both on groups of members and on the community as a whole.

To begin with, organizations must develop the capability to conduct targeted population-specific screening, followed up by wellness and health care programs for high-risk population groups. Many organizations are developing population-based care paths, which detail the frequency and kinds of screening, as well as a schedule of follow-up programs. Before reaching out to individuals, health care managers must create pro-

*Figure 15* LIFE CARE TEAMS

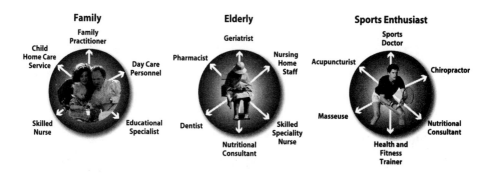

**Family**
- Family Practitioner
- Child Home Care Service
- Day Care Personnel
- Skilled Nurse
- Educational Specialist

**Elderly**
- Geriatrist
- Pharmacist
- Nursing Home Staff
- Dentist
- Skilled Speciality Nurse
- Nutritional Consultant

**Sports Enthusiast**
- Sports Doctor
- Acupuncturist
- Chiropractor
- Masseuse
- Nutritional Consultant
- Health and Fitness Trainer

grams to reach out to targeted populations, creating an awareness of risks and undertaking groupwide education. Often, the health care organization has to launch programs to stimulate interest in taking advantage of preventive services.

United HealthCare, based in Minnetonka, Minnesota, for example, sends letters to selected female plan members in a given location to encourage them to have mammography checks. Its goal is to discover breast cancer at the earliest stage, when nine out of ten women treated go on to live a healthy life, as opposed to the latest stage, when only one out of ten survive. Early treatment also costs far less: not much more than $10,000, compared with well over $100,000 for late-stage surgery and therapy. (Zablocki 1996) United has developed similar letters to encourage parents to bring children in for immunizations, and it is contemplating having nurses make phone calls and mailing follow-up letters to people at risk from congestive heart failure, diabetes, and asthma. (Zablocki 1996)

Many organizations now tailor programs for groups of employers whose workforces run similar health risks. They benefit from customized programs, which can reduce time lost from work and increase productivity. Henry Ford Health Systems, for example, is working directly with General Motors to build a health and fitness center next to GM's Detroit plants. The new center will accommodate 3,500 members, as well as Henry Ford's cardiac rehabilitation program, athletic medicine center, and full-service physical and occupational rehabilitation program. ("Integrated Health Systems" 1995) Such close cooperation with one employer allows Henry Ford Health Systems to tailor preventive services for the most common risks of a specific population.

Some innovative large employers have, in fact, taken things into their own hands in an effort to improve the overall health and productivity of their workforce. For example, Federal Express, in partnership with a physician-run demand management firm called Options and Choices, has been focused on outcomes and productivity to measure health plan value since the late 1980s. This team combined health plan data, human resource information such as performance appraisal and absenteeism, and health risk appraisal data into a single data base and developed a proprietary data mining tool to identify the most likely high-utilization segments and predict future risk. This information enabled the organizations to develop targeted strategies for disease-management programs in areas such as maternity, musculoskeletal injuries, and alcohol and drug problems, all of which have resulted in yearly health cost reductions for Federal Express at a time when many similar employers faced double-digit cost increases.

This team also developed a proactive call center that focused on high-risk individuals to reduce absenteeism and prevent disability. Coordinated referrals from these call center interactions back to the health plans improved employee health as well as satisfaction with their health plan partners. Employees have become so familiar with—and found such value in—this call center that many of them are now making calls to the center in an effort to maintain all aspects of their overall health and interact more effectively with their health care providers.

More and more employers are getting into the action because of the significance of the numbers. When items such as absenteeism, replacement worker costs, and lost productivity are factored in, the cost implications are staggering. The following data, from a survey conducted by Andersen Consulting, illustrates the magnitude of cost savings achievable through the types of proactive health management approaches described above:

▼ A $128-billion auto manufacturer: potential savings of $3–4 billion per year

▼ A $15-billion diversified high-technology manufacturer: potential savings of $450 million per year

▼ An $8-billion telecommunications company: potential savings of $400 million per year.

These are huge numbers and could significantly increase the net income and earnings per share of these organizations.

While tending to the preventive care of its own membership, winning health care organizations will also recognize the health care needs of entire communities. Many health care leaders continue to make public health programs a priority. Aside from serving charitable ends, health care organizations in the future may well find that improving community health improves their business. After all, an unhealthy community, suffering from violence, drug abuse, alcoholism, and poverty, generates a long list of tragically unnecessary health problems, often dealt with at high cost in the emergency room. While there are certainly differing views on whose responsibility it is to make it happen, a healthy community clearly helps reduce the frequency of such problems, thereby saving health care organizations a great deal in terms of money, staffing, equipment, and facilities.

In upstate New York, the Medina Memorial Hospital, the Orleans County Human Services Council, and the Medina/Albion Ministers Association have worked together to establish programs that offer free prenatal care, nutritional care, and parenting classes. The council has also launched a Regional Action Phone (RAP) that provides a 24-hour crisis hotline staffed by volunteers who take calls from abusive parents. (Rauber 1994; Sasenick 1994)

Under CEO Gail Warden, Henry Ford Health Systems offers similar programs. In 1994, Warden recognized that the organization was not reaching poor children. Securing a grant from the W.K. Kellogg Foundation of Battle Creek, Michigan, he established (in partnership with the Detroit Public Schools, the Detroit Health Department, and the Michigan Department of Public Health) clinics at thirteen inner-city middle and high schools. The clinics provide immunizations, dental hygiene, nutritional counseling, and other health care basics. ("Michigan Memo" 1994) Warden hopes the clinics will engender healthy behaviors, which the adolescents will then carry into adulthood. ("Integrated Health Systems" 1995)

Some health care executives believe so strongly in community health that they have actually linked their pay to it. A percentage of the salary of John G. O'Brien, chief executive of Cambridge Hospital, in Cambridge, Massachusetts, will be linked to measurements of the health status of the community. O'Brien actually pushed his board of directors to measure him in this fashion. (Sherer 1994) Though no organization has yet developed broadly embraced standards for community health status, O'Brien has set a course that promises to make such measures a hard reality for health care executives.

Today's hard reality, however, is that health care organizations hoping to win in the future must urgently address the issue of effectively dealing with the demand side of health care—for the individual, for at-risk population groups, and for the community as a whole. Nearly every organization budgets more these days for prevention and health. But the signal that organizations have actually transformed themselves into enterprises that emphasize the demand side will not come until they compete for consumer dollars based on their performance in preventive health, wellness, and chronic disease management.

In early 1995, Aetna showed that the changeover has begun. Aetna released figures required under the new Health Plan Employer Data Information Set (HEDIS) 2.0, which is a set of some 60 measures of performance quality, member satisfaction, membership, and finance. Administered by the National Committee for Quality Assurance, the organization that accredits HMOs, HEDIS 2.0 has rapidly become a highly visible measure of HMO performance. Aetna surpassed ambitious federal goals for childhood immunization, mammography screening, and asthma inpatient admission rates. While the federal government aims to have 90 percent of children immunized by age 2, Aetna reported a rate of 96 percent. ("Aetna Health Plans" 1995)

Kaiser Permanente Northern California Region released a 60-page report card in 1993 that details the organization's performance record in a format intended primarily for health care managers rather than consumers. A number of shorter brochures and supplements, including data on immunization rates, mammographies, vaginal births after C-sections, and laminectomies, provide information for prospective members and can be used as a recruiting tool. But Kaiser Permanente intends the full report to be a way of measuring outcomes for its own internal evaluation as well as for its competitive space. (Zablocki 1994)

Kaiser Permanente's and Aetna's accomplishments are impressive, but more important is the message that these organizations send about competition in health care. In the future, winning health care companies that surpass preventive health goals will be the rule: In managing individual and population health, they will show consumers that they are getting value for their health care dollars. As Dr. Harry P. Wetzler, director of technology and research at the Health Outcomes Institute in Bloomington, Minnesota, observes, it is essential to educate people about the limits of medical care and the kinds of outcomes they should expect, as well as to achieve consensus within the profession on evaluating outcomes as a means of improving the delivery of care. "Health care occurs primarily at the practice level between patient and practitioner," Wetzler says. "We can improve these decisions and have a better health care system by collecting data on patients, processes, and outcomes." (Wetzler 1994)

The HEDIS 2.0 measures make significant progress in addressing this need for consensus within the profession. As organizations seek to create new competitive space for themselves, they will see the benefits of developing the competency of proactively managing health delivery through such innovations as the life care plan and care teams customized for the individual or population. As we will see in the next chapter, this health care must be organized around delivering the right care in the right place at the right time by the right person. In some cases the right person can be the individual patient or member who receives the information that directs appropriate self-care. In cases of direct patient-practitioner relationships, the right care will be one of the hallmarks of winning health enterprises.

# REFERENCES

Aetna Health Plans HMO receives high marks. 1995. PRNewswire, February 27.

Burke, Terrence. 1995. Interview with Ken Jennings and Dave Blume. Washington, D.C.

Greenstone Healthcare solutions to partner with Occupational Health Strategies (OHS). 1995. PRNewswire. July 5.

Integrated health systems and delivery networks: reforming health care delivery. 1995. Unpublished working paper. Henry Ford Health System. October 26.

Michigan memo. 1994. *Detroit Free Press*, June 10, 2C.

Rauber, Chris. 1994. Communities that are making a difference. *Healthcare Forum*, July–August, 73–77.

Sasenick, Susan M. On healthier communities. May–June 1994. Supplement to *Healthcare Forum*.

Share, Andrea. 1996. Interview with Susan Vanderpool and Erik Hansen. March 4.

Sherer, Jill L. 1994. Linking incomes and outcomes. *Hospitals and Health Networks*, February 20, 39–42, 44.

Wetzler, Harry P. July–August 1994. Outcomes measurement. *Healthcare Forum* Compendium Series. 43–53.

Zablocki, Elaine. 1994. Employer report cards. *HMO Magazine*, March–April, 26–31.

————1996. Bringing prevention home. *Healthplan*, March–April, 28–35.

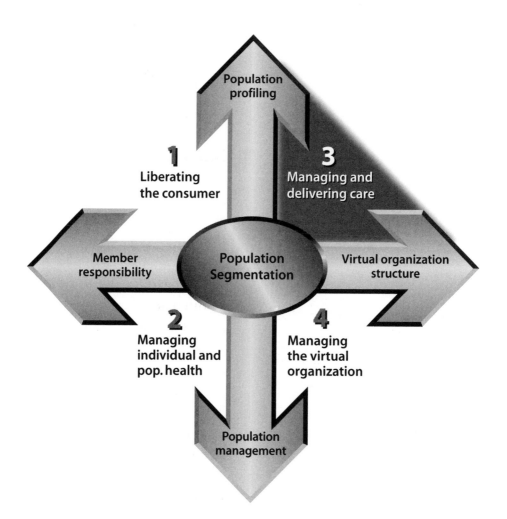

# 6

## MANAGING AND DELIVERING CARE

G ail Warden, chief executive of Henry Ford Health System in Detroit, has both bad news and good news for medical specialists. The bad news is that in the coming years the Henry Ford organization will not be needing many of them. Pediatricians, internists, and family doctors, according to Warden's plan, will appropriate a big chunk of the specialists' cases.

The good news is that the remaining specialists will no longer have to stifle their yawns when they have to deal with an endless succession of routine cases. Instead, they'll devote their time to diagnosing and treating difficult cases that demand a specialist's expertise.

Warden, like many other leaders of managed care organizations, concluded long ago that the ratio of specialists to primary care physicians was way out of whack. A workforce with two specialists for each primary care physician (a configuration typical of U.S. health care) simply costs too much and serves patients poorly. Warden aims to cast the specialists in a new role as mentors, consultants, and collaborators. ("Integrated Health" 1995)

Already, Henry Ford specialists in orthopedics, dermatology, and otolaryngology have embarked on that makeover. They have prepared new guidelines to help the primary care physicians identify the right cases to refer to specialists. As a result, they have slashed the rate of referrals and improved access to specialty care for those patients who really need it. Certain specialists in specific cases—pulmonologists who care for asthmatics and cardiologists who treat high-risk heart-disease patients—function essentially as primary care providers, eliminating the need for complex, costly, and non-value-added referral and authorization processes. ("Integrated Health" 1995)

Warden also supports programs that increase the numbers of primary care physicians. In 1994, Henry Ford, in collaboration with Cleveland's Case Western Reserve University, won a $2.4-million grant from the Robert Wood Johnson Foundation to train primary care doctors. (Santiago 1994) Warden and his staff are studying the idea of retraining specialists: They are keeping a close watch on Mercy Health and Medical Center in San Diego, the University of Tennessee, and the Medical College of Pennsylvania, all of which already have such programs. (Raphael 1994)

The case of Henry Ford shows that an upheaval lies ahead for many health care organizations. This upheaval will require organizations to build the third key competency for winning in the health care industry of the future: managing and delivering care. Organizations must revamp their plans for mobilizing, coordinating, and delivering services across the care continuum.

The overall objective of this third key competency is delivery of the right service in the right setting by the right person using the right processes. The right service implies those tests, procedures, and prescriptions indicated by best practices. The right setting means moving care routinely given by physicians in hospitals and doctors' offices to more consumer-friendly and lower-cost settings, including the consumer's home, by virtualizing many of today's location-bound services. The right person implies abandoning today's highest common denominator model of care and channeling care from high-cost specialists and physicians to other health care professionals, using teams that span various clinical settings. The right process means reengineering delivery processes to eliminate waste and inefficiency and making the most of the consumer's and care giver's time. The overall goal is to reduce costs and improve quality and service at every point of contact with the consumer.

## Primary and Specialty Care

To build a core competency in the management and delivery of health care, organizations must first reengineer primary and specialty care. Although the leaders of many health care organizations believe that they have already reengineered primary care (or, more likely, that the market has forced them to reengineer), they will find that a competitive competency in primary and specialty care requires still further transformation. Physicians, nurses, and other care providers in winning health care organizations will have to work as teams, sharing decision-making authority with assistants. Most will renegotiate the division of labor and authority between primary and specialty care and among physicians, nurses, medical assistants, and other care providers. They will also reengineer the processes of outpatient care.

As members of a team, they will examine their daily work load, limiting their attention to those tasks that add the most value. For example, in the name of efficiency—and in the name of providing value to consumers—certain tasks will be leveraged from physicians to nurse practitioners and physician extenders. A pediatrician need not see every ear infection; nurse practitioners are skilled at assessing and treating such cases, requiring consultation with pediatricians only when assessment results fall outside of normal findings. In turn, nurses, or physician assistants, can delegate routine tasks to nursing assistants and health aides. The goal is to allocate work to the care giver who can most economically deliver competent care.

The new team structure removes doctors as the essential link in the chain of every consumer's care. To serve some members with diabetes, for example, physicians can share care responsibilities with a team comprising a nurse, a pharmacist, and a dietitian. The team would provide care that is not only economical but also the appropriate level for each situation. Those teams, or their members, would serve each consumer across the continuum of care, from doctor's office to hospital to skilled nursing facility to home care.

This new structure will continue to move primary care physicians from traditional gatekeeper roles to roles of health care coaches and facilitators. As consumers continue to gain increasing access to previously restricted medical and clinical information, the structure will also move physicians to act as "personal health navigators," who help patients obtain and use information in the most correct manner. If traditional health plans and providers do not assume this new role, new market entrants will fill the gap. For example, consumers can already hire American Medical Consumers, a firm recently launched by physician Vincent Riccardi, to review their cases and work with their physicians to obtain appropriate care.

In addition to role changes, physicians will also need to find ways to effectively utilize and integrate phone triage services and encourage safe but aggressive self-care when and where appropriate. Some physicians are even developing their own phone services that, when appropriate, substitute fee calls for office visits. In short, with the help of well-trained, leveraged staff and the appropriate support tools and enablers, many physicians can significantly increase the size of their panels (fixed groups of patients) and improve service levels and quality of care.

In the same way that winning organizations must encourage primary care physicians to leverage their skills, they must encourage specialists to spend their time where they add greatest value. Specialists will in many cases relinquish routine cases to primary care physicians. In an effort to better serve population segments, on the other hand, some specialists will take on expanded primary care and contact roles for selected groups. The ultimate goal is for all providers—primary care physicians, specialists, nurse practitioners, and so on—to focus on specific member segments and activities where they can add the greatest overall value.

Like many leading health care organizations, Henry Ford Health System uses teams of physicians, nurses, physician assistants, and technicians to care for panels of patients. In addition to improving service quality and patient satisfaction, the several member teams assure that patients receive prompt attention. Meanwhile, physicians have more time to handle complex cases. ("Integrated Health" 1995)

Organizations that do not make the shift to team care will find themselves at a distinct disadvantage. During a preliminary opportunity assessment, one staff model HMO found that, according to physicians, 52 percent of customer visits could be handled by nonphysicians. This assumes other appropriate health care delivery personnel were available and effectively trained, and patient preferences were met. Twenty percent of visits to physician assistants, nurse practitioners, and other midlevel care givers could be handled by nurses given similar conditions. This organization concluded that broadening the roles of midlevel providers, nurses, and the members themselves could provide significant savings for the company and its members. Additionally, the company concluded it could save even more by cross-training staff, redefining the role of physicians and specialists, and designating alternate team members to help with certain tasks.

To facilitate change in the way they work, specialists and primary care physicians will establish demand management guidelines, aligning them with care path guidelines. For example, certain conditions will be preapproved for referrals and treatments. The goal is to develop a consistent, coordinated referral system in concert with all stakeholders while eliminating much of the paperwork and handoffs that typify traditional utilization management. A preliminary study indicates that more than 50 percent of current manual interventions could be eliminated if appropriate preapprovals were implemented.

The HMO's analysis also indicates the magnitude of other benefits that could result from improved automation and workflows. In the analysis of its documentation processes, for example, the company found that physician documentation can cost up to $4.5 million per year. Its evaluation of nursing identified a potential 13 percent increase in productivity that could be achieved by reducing administrative rework. The room for improvement—and the risk to the organization's competitiveness—was huge.

The HMO, therefore, proposed a number of ways to streamline work processes. The company plans to simplify forms, establish a number of shortcuts for completing those forms, and install an integrated electronic medical record. By establishing guidelines through statistical sampling techniques, the number of referrals that require authorization will be lowered, further reducing paperwork, manual interventions, and costs while improving customer satisfaction. The company will assure that each step contributes to the consumer's experience, minimizing the number of times information, people, or supplies are passed from one person to another.

Although many physicians at the HMO (and elsewhere) often feel beleaguered by all the forces for change, the conceptual tables are turning in their favor. The surest sign of this reversal is the meteoric growth of physician practice management companies like MedPartners of Birmingham, Alabama. On track to grow up to 40 percent per year, MedPartners buys physician practices, injecting its capital and installing management practices and information systems to help physicians deliver outstanding care and service. Larry House, MedPartners' chairman and CEO, recognizes that health care excellence will depend on physicians' ability to transfer freely but prudently the maximum possible amount of knowledge, expertise, compassion, and hands-on care to the people they serve. "The physician is being brought into focus as the manager of care," says House. "The insurance company can't manage that care. The hospitals can't manage that care." (House 1995)

Physicians will be called on to manage care according to best-practice standards. They will have to take advantage of evidence-based clinical guidelines, lifetime and episodic care paths, online medical references, and both population-based and individual-outcomes research. Additionally, they will have to employ new information technology tools and quality management practices that will help them continuously improve outcomes and consumer satisfaction. Along with changes such as these, physicians will reestablish ownership of their work, playing an important new role in the information-intensive, consumer-driven health care world of the future.

MedPartners plans to accomplish the changeover in part by having all physicians accept some form of risk such as capitation (a fixed fee per patient) over the long term. Risk incentives are intended to motivate doctors to improve the health of their members and minimize long-term costs through a focused approach to wellness, prevention, and disease management. The idea, according to House, is that physicians will devise systems and mechanisms to reduce interactions and improve the surveillance of each consumer's health. "We want to empower, lead, and teach physicians to manage care in the way that is best for the patient. It is a massive revolution," House says. "There will be winners and losers economically, but if you can recast your role appropriately and realign your relationships, you can be a winner. Those that try to hang onto the old and not adapt to the new will be hurt." (House 1995)

### Hospital Care

Perhaps no process in health care has received as much attention as care delivery to ailing patients. Because so much of that attention is due to concern about the high cost of inpatient care, many health care organizations are developing sophisticated ways to reduce the need to hospitalize people in the first place. For those who do require acute inpatient services, health care enterprises must find more effective ways to deliver care.

Since the late 1980s, hospitals everywhere have been reengineering care delivery. Early efforts sought to create patient-focused care, the principles and practices of which, although no longer new, are the foundation of today's far-reaching programs to reengineer care across the continuum.

The basic premise of patient-focused care is that by reorganizing hospital services around the needs of the patient, versus functional departments and professions, organizations can achieve quantum improvements in cost, quality, and service. In the past, hospitals assumed that specialization would boost quality through repetition of tasks and that centralization would lower costs through higher utilization rates and economies of scale. While these are valid assumptions to some extent, both operating principles have been taken to counterproductive extremes. Today, hospitals practicing patient-focused care group patients with similar clinical needs into larger, more homogeneous patient care centers. In addition to reducing costs, this reaggregation improves the ability to better match staff and services with patients. (Miller 1994)

Patient-focused care units let hospitals follow a second principle of patient-focused care: redeployment, in which the hospital moves many departmental services nearer to the patient. Before the advent of patient-focused care, a patient at the Medical Center in Beaver, Pennsylvania, could expect to travel almost two miles in the course of a six-day stay for tests alone. In the early 1990s, when Beaver began reengineering, it grouped patients into nine units and moved 80 percent of services, including admissions, housekeeping, phlebotomy, electrocardiography, and respiratory therapy, from central departments to unit-based providers. The pharmacy, labs, and X-ray services relocated into multiple satellite units closer to each unit. Now patients spend more time in their rooms and less time rolling down the hallways. (Taylor 1994; Blocker, Lorenz, and Schartner 1994)

Effective patient-focused care also depends on a hospital

staff with a broad range of skills, a principle that reverses the decades-long narrowing of employees' roles. Today's complex health care processes demand multiskilled personnel. Nurses, for example, are expanding their roles to take on phlebotomy, electrocardiography, nutrition, and other clinical, administrative, and support activities. They are also enhancing their skills in traditional areas of care-giving.

In many patient-focused care hospitals, a single multi-skilled worker draws blood and starts intravenous injections, tasks that in the past required two specialists. Both Lee Memorial Hospital in Fort Myers, Florida, and the Medical Center in Beaver, Pennsylvania, have consolidated job descriptions to encourage staff members to develop several areas of expertise. Those hospitals have slashed the number of handoffs in many of their processes, sharply reduced the chance for errors, and boosted patient satisfaction by trimming the number of staff members each patient encounters. According to Terry Biss, senior vice president of the Medical Center, "Patients were seeing as many as 70 different people during a hospital stay." (Qtd. in Taylor 1994) Patients feel that a smaller, core group of staff gives more attentive care.

Recent revelations that hospitals have committed errors in dispensing medication demonstrate other risks inherent in narrow specialization. The frequent handoffs and the notion that health care quality depends on well-trained people who never make errors often lead to the worst possible outcomes. Lucian Leape of the Harvard School of Public Health estimates that, in the United States alone, 180,000 people die each year in part as a result of hospital errors. That death toll is equal to the toll of three jumbo jet crashes every two days. ("Reducing the Incidence" 1995)

As we saw in Chapter 5, care teams are an important part of reengineering care delivery processes. As with primary and specialty care, teams of multiskilled professionals take responsibility for each patient, and the hospital can reduce the number of people who work with each patient. The teams also lower labor costs by reducing the 20 to 25 percent of idle time typical of workers whose jobs are narrowly defined.

The fifth principle of patient-focused care is exception-based care management, which comprises care protocols, or clinical paths, and charting by exception. With standard protocols, physicians, nurses, and other care givers can note the completion of standard tasks that meet expected outcomes with a simple tick mark, making detailed notes only for exceptions rather than for every element of care.

Together, care protocols and charting by exception can expedite hospital care, increase quality, and dramatically reduce the time staff spend on paperwork. In a 1995 Andersen Consulting survey, 81 percent of hospitals reported using care protocols, and 77 percent reported using charting by exception. Care protocols and charting by exception are most commonly applied to coronary bypasses, but many hospitals have also developed paths for scores of other ailments, such as pneumonia, hysterectomies, urinary tract infections, and eating disorders. People responding to the Andersen survey cited various benefits of clinical paths, from decreased lengths of stay and decreased costs to improved multidisciplinary teamwork and communication. ("New Survey" 1995)

A sixth principle of patient-focused care is realignment of authority, accountability, and management structures. As hospitals have reengineered, they have reworked their hierarchies and performance indicators. When teams in patient care units take responsibility for patient care, authority begins to shift from functional department directors to care center leaders. Accordingly, performance measures shift from those monitoring departmental efficiency to those monitoring patient service and care center effectiveness. Patient-focused care units emphasize greater satisfaction and a shorter length of stay. At the Medical Center, for example, patient-focused care shortened the average length of stay from 6.4 days in 1993 to 5.2 days by May 1994. (Blocker, Lorenz, and Schartner 1994)

### Cross-Continuum Care

Applying the principles of patient-focused care to inpatient care delivery has yielded remarkable cost savings and sharply higher quality and consumer satisfaction ratings. Cost savings have typically ranged from 10 percent to 15 percent, topping out at 28 percent. But as successful as patient-focused strategies have been inside hospitals, they offer far more significant potential when applied across the continuum of care, especially when they focus on eliminating the need for hospitalization. (Miller 1994)

As organizations bring preventive, outpatient, inpatient, rehabilitative, and long-term care under one organizational roof—whether vertical or virtual—they can readily apply the principle of reaggregation across the care continuum. The regrouping of patients and services to match consumer and community needs enables the organization to consolidate various administrative, clinical, and support services within the system. For example, organizations can establish centers of excellence for technology-intensive services such as cardiac surgery and joint replacements.

Grant Medical Center in Columbus, Ohio, has become an orthopedic center of excellence offering joint replacements to members of the emerging U.S. Healthcorp system. Grant has created longitudinal care paths that encompass the surgeon's office, hospital, skilled nursing facility, and patient's home. The organization has also vertically integrated its work with that of its partners and suppliers such as implant manufacturers. It uses cross-continuum teams to provide care as the patient moves from the hospital to the rehab center to home. Team members are cross-trained to provide care across multiple settings, practicing principles of exception-based care management. (Lorenz 1995)

Organizations that reengineer across the continuum will realize that they are essentially designing a new care delivery and network architecture. They are applying the redeployment principles by redistributing and relocating various services across the care continuum, from prevention and wellness services through hospice care. That distribution will give consumers a choice of such traditional settings as physician offices and hospitals, as well as such nontraditional settings as offices, factories, and community centers.

As an example, Henry Ford Health System created a program called Center for Senior Independence. The center uses a multidisciplinary approach, combining medical services, transportation, and social services to care for the elderly in their homes. The goal is to avoid institutionalization of the elderly who are unable to manage multiple health problems.

Many organizations are already applying the principle of case coordination across the continuum of care. For example, at Brookwood Medical Center in Birmingham, Alabama, twenty laptop-toting specialty nurses create a care plan for all hospital patients, tracking their progress and following up after they leave the hospital. Follow-up can last as long as a year in the cases of diabetics. In addition, those nurses participate in admissions, utilization review, social work, and discharge planning. (Blocker, Lorenz, and Schartner 1994)

The life care paths discussed in Chapter 5 can also be useful tools for case coordination. Nurses and other members of ad hoc teams charged with the care of individual patients could rely on life care software to track and manage not only such conditions as diabetes but other health risks and chronic conditions as well. Powerful information technology will provide care givers with the entire collection of care paths—preventive, chronic disease, episodic—and health information for each consumer's lifetime of care.

## Performance Management

To support these changes in care delivery and management, winning health care enterprises must build enhanced capabilities in performance measurement. Reliable facts and figures about current performance form the basis for improving primary, specialty, and hospital care. At Henry Ford Health System, for example, members regularly complete satisfaction surveys and participate in focus groups. Working with care givers, analysts compare the data with national benchmarks and develop tactics for improving performance.

Quality management has topped the agenda of CEO Gail Warden since early in the decade. Warden stresses that a disciplined, data-based approach forms the foundation for creating and operating a high-quality organization. Henry Ford focuses on cycles of continuous improvement, empowering employees and teams to make better decisions. In addition, it fosters systems thinking, taking a broad view of complex organizational processes to find innovative solutions to problems. Perhaps the most powerful aspect of quality management in health care organizations is its creation of consumer mindedness: the will and the ability to understand and deliver what the health care consumer wants. ("Integrated Health" 1995)

Several years ago, the managers of Henry Ford discovered that, as in many places, consumers were dissatisfied with their visits to their primary care physicians. Few identified with one doctor; most shopped around for appointments. They reported that the phone system was hard to use. Furthermore, inadequate access to specialty care frustrated them, and they reported that the quality of triage and phone advice varied significantly from office to office.

To improve patient visits, staff from the Henry Ford Medical Group dissected the process. The staff developed step-by-step performance measures that traced the process from the time the consumer placed the initial call to the checkout. Those measures included such basics as phone call abandonment rates, time spent in waiting rooms, time spent with physicians, and lead times for appointments with specialists. By better understanding the process, measuring key points of performance, and devising solutions to rectify problems, Henry Ford's management expects to boost consumer satisfaction at primary care offices. (Anctil and Blazar 1994)

Managing performance through measurement is also important in improving hospital care. At the top level, the goal may be simply to improve the quality of care by reducing variation. Top-level outcomes measures might include length of hospital stay, readmission rates, and number of complications. These measures are supported by process measures that contribute to outcomes, such as the percentage of time clinical guidelines are used or the percentage of patients that deviate from a clinical path.

The power of measurements to guide improvement makes them essential to competitiveness. Consider that in 1992 Bethany Hospital in Chicago began to measure the length of hospital stays for adult asthma patients and track how often they returned to the emergency room or to inpatient care. Finding that the revisit rate was an unsatisfactory 11.6 percent, Bethany reviewed its process for handling asthmatics. A team of physicians studied clinical data and compared Bethany's emergency-room and inpatient protocols with those of the National Institutes of Health's Consensus Conference Report. The team reworked its protocols, beefed up education for patients and families, developed a new information system to track patients, and instituted regular pulmonary function testing. By 1995, the asthmatic emergency room revisit rate had plunged below 3 percent. ("Storyboard: Adult Asthma" 1995)

As organizations extend their coordination across the continuum, performance measurement will become increasingly important. New measures will have to include a variety of system-level indicators, all of which dovetail with local measures of primary, specialty, and hospital care. Taken together, the data from multiple levels of measurement provides the factual basis for a systemwide learning organization.

### The Information Technology Advantage

A powerful aid to the transformation of care across all settings is information technology. One particularly important capability is moving information down the professional ladder, from specialists to primary care physicians, physicians' assistants and nurses, and even consumers. Given that most consumers have only routine health worries, care givers other than the physician can handle most inquiries. Consumers themselves can obtain answers to their concerns with the help of a variety of new systems for medical information, diagnosis, and advice. For example, many health organizations now provide videos to parents to help them understand how best to care for a feverish child. Care givers have learned that even such simple technology can cut the number of pediatric visits by as much as 35 percent. (Medical Leadership Council 1995)

The potential for online self-help and self-diagnosis software is even greater, especially as health care organizations make it possible for consumers to conduct electronic conversations with their care givers. As we shall see in the next chapter, triage nurses in particular are helping to reduce the number of unnecessary visits to primary care physicians and emergency rooms.

Information technology also facilitates automated appointment scheduling and electronic referral authorization. An online appointment scheduling system could follow the organization's scheduling rules while providing convenient access for consumers. It could also track appointments, automatically issuing confirmations and reminders. The referral system would automatically verify coverage, authorize appointments, and alert specialists when new appointments are scheduled.

Perhaps the most important use of information technology in transforming care and service delivery will be the automation of the life care plans discussed in Chapter 5. Life care plan software will generate standard preventive, chronic disease, and episodic care paths for treatment of a range of common ailments. Providers can tailor the paths for each patient based on individual medical history, symptoms, vital signs, and other data, which then structure subsequent clinical and administrative activity. Such a system will give physicians, nurses, and other authorized care givers a reliable tool for excellent care and service, whether during primary care, specialty care, hospital care, or postacute care.

Although many changes have already swept through the industry, they are only the beginning. Future software integrated with life care plans will automatically suggest orders and treatments. Care-management tools will enable nurses, physicians, and case managers to review online every detail of a patient's case, evaluate the care, and document family history. These systems will also link administrative applications, allowing access to coverage provisions, billing, and claims.

Flowing throughout the system, the information from exception-based charting and other procedures will feed outcomes systems, reveal variances from standard practice, and identify opportunities for improvement. Ultimately, the life care tool and associated software will become the central focus of care delivery and management.

Henry Ford Health System has laid the foundation for such a system with its innovative Medical Information Management system, which integrates clinical and patient data through a common interface. With this system, physicians can call up information about any patient's care—lab results, X-rays, appointments—from any Henry Ford Health System location. ("Integrated Health" 1995) The organization is also developing a Patient Care Referral system to help providers handle electronically such tasks as referrals, precertification, claims submission, and appointment scheduling.

Now in development by a number of health plans, delivery systems, and pharmaceutical companies, clinical data repositories and data warehouses will capture and store information on clinical processes in primary, specialty, and hospital settings. Henry Ford Health System, for example, is creating a forerunner of a broad clinical repository, which it calls the Corporate Data Store, to integrate clinical work with financial and demographic data. Used for such tasks as health services research, clinical effectiveness research, and clinical guideline creation, this data store is the basis for continuous improvement. ("Integrated Health" 1995)

United HealthCare is another example of an organization that has truly capitalized on its information technology capabilities to improve care delivery processes across its plan and provider networks. A key enabler of this success has been a robust back-end data warehousing capability from which United is able to extract useful medical management information from claims. For example, based on pharmacy claims data coupled with previous encounter information, they can determine that a member with diabetes is not refilling her prescriptions as often as she would if she were following the optimal diabetic care path. Armed with this information, case managers can notify the members' primary care physician, who can follow up directly with the member before an adverse event, such as a preventable hospitalization, occurs. (Anderson 1996)

Several major health plans are also investigating sophisticated customer information systems that will incorporate selected clinical and administrative information as well as data such as health risk assessment results. These systems will improve customer service far beyond what today's health plans typically provide. Through these systems, tomorrow's care givers will have all the relevant information for managing care, service, and member contact across the continuum and throughout a member's life.

## *Virtualizing Care Delivery*

Colusa Community Hospital, a 56-bed health care facility in rural Colusa, California, could not afford to hire a full-time radiologist, but it could afford a $10,000 off-the-shelf computer equipped with a modem. With the new technology, the hospital provides complete radiology services by using regular phone lines to connect to a radiology group in Chico, 50 miles away. With that computer link, Colusa physicians are now able to resume obstetric services, a practice discontinued by the hospital in 1987. Online specialists at the University of California Medical Center at Davis observe women in labor. In emergencies, some women have been airlifted via helicopter to Sacramento. (Robertson 1995)

Successful telemedicine requires collaboration. To deliver new or better health care services, the winning health care enterprise will have to stay alert to the potential of innovative partnerships. One public hospital in Corpus Christi, Texas, has contracted with HEB Grocery, a supermarket with a pharmacy, to give care to diabetics. The hospital pays the pharmacy each time patients receive a 90-minute assessment, group education, and a 30-minute follow-up consultation with a pharmacist. A physician must sign off on the arrangement, which allows the pharmacy to sell prescriptions to the diabetics and direct them to appropriate foods in the HEB grocery aisles. ("Chains and Business" 1995)

Park Medical Center in Columbus, Ohio, is now partnered with American Transitional Hospitals of Franklin, Tennessee, which will offer respiratory and other therapy to help gravely ill patients learn to breathe without ventilators. The company reports that its services cost 30 to 60 percent less than those offered by traditional hospitals. (Selis 1995)

Information technology, including telemedicine, and organizational collaboration are two ways of virtualizing care delivery and providing value to customers across the continuum of care. As we will see in Chapter 7, the virtual organization will expand the capabilities of any single enterprise through technology and strategic partnerships.

### Care Management and Administration

To boost customer satisfaction and improve efficiency, winning health enterprises are also reengineering their other member touch points, including administrative processes such as appointment scheduling, customer service, claims, and billing.

Appointment scheduling influences both the level of service delivered to the consumer and the efficient use of health care professionals' time. For the consumer, the organization must provide easy access to visits, procedures, and services in all locations and in all departments. It should also organize scheduling to coordinate visits across the continuum, issue prompts and follow-up reminders, and allow patients to schedule their own preventive care.

We have all been on the receiving end of bad service and recognize that few things in life can be so frustrating and irritating. In many health care organizations service to consumers remains disjointed: A customer telephones for advice or information, and the call is bounced from one representative to another. Consumers often receive inconsistent service depending on the time, nature, and recipient of their calls. As organizations expand their offerings in products and services, consumer dissatisfaction is bound to increase unless these enterprises follow the example of industries such as lodging, mail order, and financial services, which have distinguished themselves by delivering excellent service.

HealthPartners of Minneapolis has made it a goal to provide caring, efficient, and effective services for all customers and to drive a process that continuously improves those services. HealthPartners representatives seek to accomplish three objectives: to resolve all inquiries directly without phone transfer; to give professional, caring service by taking ownership of the problems raised by each customer; and to make basic information available 24 hours a day. In reengineering customer service, HealthPartners now centralizes its customer service operations. Integrated computer and telephone systems prioritize and distribute calls. Voice-recognition technology permits round-the-clock service coverage. HealthPartners representatives capture complete customer contact information at workstations, use work flow technology to manage casework, and rely on a customer service database to store all necessary data. When needed, special consultants in billing, enrollment, and medical management stand by to help frontline representatives. Through such innovations, representatives can provide fast, consistent information.

Organizations will improve customer service even more by integrating clinical and administrative information and processes. Andersen Consulting has developed a call center prototype to illustrate this point. In one scenario, when a consumer calls with a question about a claim or payment, the customer service representative in the call center is prompted to check the member's life care plan. The care plan alerts the representative that the member is overdue for a PAP smear or a mammogram. Passing a polite reminder on to the member of the need to schedule the test is an example of the proactive, courteous service that will become ever more important to health care enterprises' competitiveness.

There are probably fewer ways to make the billing process more palatable to consumers, but a good start is to make it efficient and accurate. HealthPartners has started to improve this process by reengineering its entire revenue management cycle, from determination of eligibility to billing, to collection and management of receivables. At HealthPartners, managers seek to maximize revenue collection by offering a billing process that customers can understand, one that is complete, consistent, and accurate. In addition, the organization increases value by responding to billing inquiries and complaints and by giving consumers itemized billing information on demand. As an innovator in the industry, HealthPartners is following the lead of world-class receivables practices in companies inside and outside the health care industry. It is launching initiatives to improve its billing process by, among other things, centralizing receivables, establishing partnerships for electronic exchange of billing documents (via electronic data interchange), and building systems that automatically calculate billing adjustments. A centralized accounts receivable department will assure smooth interfaces to the general ledger, centralize collections and statement production, and generate financial reports. As HealthPartners implements the changes, the organization expects to reap such benefits as accurate and timely billing, increased cash flow, and less delay in payments. The process will also generate a wealth of data for managing finances, speeding quality improvement programs, and supporting simplified claims processing.

In managing claims, most health care organizations today continue to rely on paper-based processes, with manual data entry and archaic systems to identify excessive, fraudulent, or incorrect claims. In addition to inaccurate payments and loss of time required to correct mistakes, these outdated systems provide inconsistent information to consumers on their coverage and poor reports to management.

At HealthPartners, managers have attacked these problems by reengineering the process of managing funds disbursement. Care givers provide detailed information to the claims personnel, who then determine coverage for authorized services according to contract terms. The goal is to determine member coverage, capture and validate information about care delivered in all settings, and reimburse correctly. HealthPartners seeks to create a process without hassles or surprises, a system with consistent, timely information that spells value for consumers.

In reengineering its funds disbursement process, Health-Partners has adopted world-class practices. It now automates the adjudication of claims, uses sophisticated reporting to prevent fraud, assures consistent reimbursement information before and after care, and creates paperless processing that includes feedback loops for continuous improvement. As the organization has reengineered funds disbursement, it has benefited from greater accuracy, less manual intervention, lower administration costs, and faster turnaround times.

In the future, winning health care organizations will try to dispense with the bulk of claims and billing altogether. Much of the delay in claims processing today stems from complex provider contracts and from referral and authorization requirements. The introduction of care paths with built-in referral and authorization protocols, however, will permit exception-based claims processing, simplifying or eliminating much of the red tape. Early evidence suggests that health plans will move away from tight control and punitive management of providers; instead, they will share incentives and accountability. The work associated with processing claims will shrink dramatically. Although the notion of invoice-free payment is still foreign to most health care enterprises, the concept is spreading rapidly in other industries.

Health care enterprises that expect to win in the future must try to watch and match the innovations cropping up elsewhere. As hotels, consumer goods companies, car rental firms, and other companies deliver superior administrative performance, consumers will expect the same from health care organizations. With that challenge in mind, HealthPartners compares its performance with that of other companies considered the best in delivering service. HealthPartners' comparisons showed, for example, that world-class companies resolve 90 to 95 percent of complaints in a single contact and that they take, on average, seven days to resolve formal complaints. Accordingly, HealthPartners has set targets approaching or equaling the best.

The challenge of managing and delivering world-class health care is imposing. Although Henry Ford Health System is a preeminent example of an integrated health enterprise, even it feels the heat of competition. In 1995, for the first time in the organization's history, CEO Gail Warden received letters from three of the organization's biggest customers—Ford Motor Company, General Motors, and Chrysler Corporation—requesting lower rates. Blue Care Network, a competitor, was charging a per-member-per-month rate that undercut Henry Ford's rate by $10. Not hesitant to admit that his organization fell short of market demands, Warden launched a three-year program to redesign all aspects of care delivery from quality management and clinical reform to decentralizing services. ("Integrated Health" 1995) And he vowed to cut $200 million in costs. (Warden 1995)

As the example of Henry Ford Health System clearly shows, even a national leader cannot afford to sit still. Health care enterprises that expect to win in the future will have to innovate continuously to manage and deliver the best care possible, learning how to take appropriate measures of their processes and promises.

# REFERENCES

Anctil, Beth, and James Blazar. 1994. Improving access to ambulatory care: linking customer judgments and performance measures. Unpublished report. Henry Ford Medical Group. Detroit, Mich.

Anderson, James. 1996. Interview with the authors. June.

Blocker, Ann, Janet Lorenz, and Carl Schartner. 1994. Care delivery reengineering: an industrial look. *Restructuring healthcare delivery: a compendium on patient-focused care.* Supplement to *The Healthcare Forum.*

Chains and business: food chain, hospital team up to offer seamless diabetic care. 1995. *Drug Topics*, May 22, 67.

House, Larry. 1995. Interview with the authors. December.

Integrated health systems and delivery networks: reforming health care delivery. 1995. Henry Ford Health System Working Paper. October 26.

Lorenz, Janet. 1995. Interview with the authors. December.

Medical Leadership Council. 1995. The new American medicine: survey of clinical reform at the frontier. Washington, D.C.: The Advisory Board.

Miller, Kurt. 1994. A look into the future: the next wave of care delivery re-engineering. *Restructuring healthcare delivery: a compendium on patient-focused care.* Supplement to *The Healthcare Forum.*

New survey reveals growing importance of clinical paths: boosting quality of care and cost-effectiveness cited as key benefits. 1995. Unpublished report. Andersen Consulting. December 5.

Raphael, Steve. 1994. Medicine seeking family values. *Crains Detroit Business,* April 25, 1.

Reducing the incidence of adverse drug events. [Interview with Lucian Leape]. 1995. *Quality connection: news from the Institute for Healthcare Improvement* 4.2 (Spring): 5–7.

Robertson, Kathy. 1995. Telemedicine rings up high hopes. *Business Journal-Sacramento,* June 19, 15.

Santiago, Raquel. 1994. CWRU receives 3-year grant to train primary physicians. *Crains Cleveland Business,* June 27, 25.

Selis, Sara. 1995. Firm to open "hospital within a hospital" at Park [Medical Center]. *Business First-Columbus,* July 3, 5.

Storyboard: adult asthma ER returns and admissions. 1995. *Quality connection: news from the Institute for Healthcare Improvement* 4.2 (Spring): 10–11.

Taylor, Susan. 1994. The Medical Center takes proactive approach to healthcare reform. *Industrial Engineering,* January, 20–23.

Warden, Gail. 1995. Interview with Ken Jennings and Kedrick Adkins. November 20.

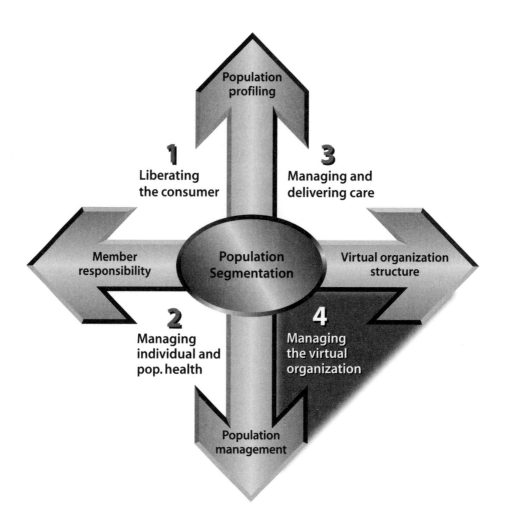

Population
profiling

**1**
Liberating
the consumer

**3**
Managing and
delivering care

Member
responsibility

Population
Segmentation

Virtual organization
structure

**2**
Managing
individual and
pop. health

**4**
Managing
the virtual
organization

Population
management

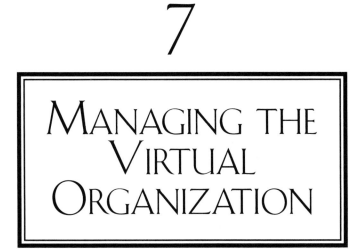

# 7

# MANAGING THE VIRTUAL ORGANIZATION

W alk into the executive offices of PacifiCare Health Systems in Cypress, California, and you'll hear people like Sam Ho, vice president, Health Services, talking about the value equation: "Value," says Ho, "equals quality of health, quality of service, and efficiency—divided by cost." Ho maintains that most organizations still focus largely on cost. PacifiCare, on the other hand, looks at the whole equation. (Ho 1995)

Ho readily admits, however, that PacifiCare cannot, alone, excel in simultaneously maximizing each of the three variables in the value equation's numerator while minimizing the cost variable in the denominator. PacifiCare could try to buy physician practices, for example, to help it come up with better results. Those physicians could supplement PacifiCare's existing care competencies. But PacifiCare, like many other organizations, simply cannot spare the capital to go shopping on such a grand scale. "We figured out that we cannot afford the vertical integration," says Ho. (Ho 1995)

So PacifiCare has instead put its faith in virtual integration. For starters, that means that it has backed away from short-term provider contracts. In 1995, the company took the unusual step of signing long-term contacts with almost all its Southern California medical groups. Whereas most HMO physician contracts run for a single year, PacifiCare drafted contracts that run at least five years, with some running up to ten. (Woodyard 1995) The long-term contracts bind PacifiCare and physicians together more tightly. Now, performance standards address not only costs but quality and resource management as well. (Ho 1995)

PacifiCare and seven of its closest provider organizations have recently launched joint programs to improve service and clinical quality. One of those programs aims to identify and develop the services purchasers demand. A second intends to develop health care education curricula tailored to member needs, and a third focuses on members' access to care and specialty referrals. (Ho 1995)

To demonstrate its interest in collaborating closely with its virtual partners, PacifiCare has established member services departments in the offices of one of its medical groups. "We reduce the general and administrative expenses, reduce the redundancy, reengineer some of the core processes," says Ho, "so we can maximize value to the customers." (Ho 1995) PacifiCare has also supplied support to its key physician partners in the areas of resource management techniques and outcomes reporting feedback.

Such innovation demonstrates that winning health care organizations will result from simultaneous change across organizational boundaries. Health care enterprises must constantly and consistently improve the experience and quality of health care across the continuum by developing this fourth key competency.

Developing and managing the virtual organization calls for integrating management practices both within and across enterprises to deliver consistent, high-value service to purchasers and consumers across the continuum of care. The virtual organization must address clinical guidelines and care path development, management of supply and demand, and development of strong relationships among purchaser, provider, and supplier.

### The Imperative of Integrated Management

One simple fact is that few health care enterprises can make it on their own. Every organization that aims to deliver seamless service across the continuum must work with at least a handful of partners. That means that all health care executives, in big organizations and small, have to figure out what kinds of partnerships are right for them.

One of the more obvious ways to build an organization is to acquire other companies. That, of course, requires capital. Many health care enterprises have taken this route, buying all the services across the health plan delivery network in the continuum, including product development, marketing and financial risk management, and care delivery. Likewise, many of these organizations have discovered that integrating all those acquired pieces into a seamlessly functional organization can consume significant time and resources.

Many enterprises, even those with adequate capital, will find that an unattractive strategy. After all, no organization, however big, can offer consumers everything. We believe that many organizations will join large networks of independent enterprises. Those networks will work as an integrated entity to provide all services. They will gain the competitive edge through virtual integration. As they do, they will discover the advantage of partnership without ownership. The networked organization can quickly change direction and restructure to meet new consumer or business demands.

PacifiCare is a good example. Through virtual integration, it has expanded across the United States from its California base. In late 1994, for example, the company formed a joint Medicare venture with Tufts Health Plan in New England. As a part of that venture, Tufts acquired PacifiCare's expertise in building a Medicare HMO. PacifiCare, on the other hand, acquired a more diverse revenue stream while entering a new market—with substantially lower risk than going it alone. (Kroll et al. 1995) PacifiCare has entered another partnership to extend its coverage from six states (California, Florida, Oklahoma, Oregon, Texas, and Washington) to 46 states. Instead of building a nationwide medical network from the ground up, the company signed a contract with Affordable Medical Networks, a unit of Health Care Compare, which runs a physician practice network of 125,000 care givers and 1,700 hospitals nationwide. (Olmos 1994)

Health care organizations can benefit from virtual integration only if they first clarify their current—as well as their desired—positions within the evolving health care system. Those positions (current and future) are functions of their competencies, people, capital, market positions, and locations. With those assessments, they must articulate clearly their objectives and strategies. Managers must determine the competitive battles they will wage on their own and those they will bypass. Partnerships will fill in the gaps.

The virtual alliance strategy has illuminated a looming issue that all health industry organizations must face: Their roles and value propositions are changing dramatically. Health insurers, for example, will have to rethink their roles in the industry and then leverage their strengths to remain successful in the future. For many years, insurers had limited their business to administering health benefit plans. With the advent of managed care, many have tried to reposition themselves as managers of care and information. They have assembled provider networks and the tools to standardize clinical practices and control utilization, but they have discovered that they have not managed care as well as some sophisticated groups of doctors. A 1995 study of six big physician-run medical groups on the West Coast showed that doctors who are paid under fixed-fee contracts do a much better job of managing utilization and costs than insurance companies. (Manley 1995)

The insurers, as they watch physician groups tackle the jobs of clinical management, utilization management, and demand management, must reassess their roles. Some are deriving the most benefit from leveraging their skills in marketing, administration, bill collection and management, information management, and building strong relationships with payers and providers. Building on their ability to connect members and providers, they may also position themselves in a new role as information integrators and interaction facilitators. That is, they will link directly with consumers and guide them through the virtual system for optimal health outcomes. In this role, they are also positioned to strengthen their brand names, as well as to develop new products for direct sales to consumers.

Any winning health care enterprise of the future must evaluate each of its services to determine which should be the pillars of their business. After they eliminate peripheral services, they can focus on those products and services based on the organization's bedrock core competencies—competencies that the organization can leverage to give the consumer ever-increasing value.

A good example of a company that has narrowed the focus

of its sharply defined competencies is Nashville-based PhyCor, a physician practice–management company. PhyCor buys the assets of physician practices and signs long-term contracts with the doctors to run those practices. PhyCor then installs its cost accounting, administrative, and medical management systems. It brings state-of-the-art management to the operation of physicians' practices, running day-to-day administration, negotiating contracts with suppliers and HMOs, and helping physicians to identify and adopt emerging best practices.

PhyCor establishes a clear role in the larger, virtual network. "We keep before our people the strategic vision on one sheet of paper," says Joe Hutts, PhyCor chief executive. "We have repeatedly said to HMOs that we don't want to be an HMO. The physician piece is the part that is going to create the value."

Hutts has worked hard to assure that PhyCor's operations mesh smoothly with those of other enterprises. On the one hand, he has invested heavily to strengthen PhyCor's most important competency: medical management. On the other, he strives to identify how PhyCor's skills either overlap or complement those of other organizations. He is committed to PhyCor's role as one piece within larger networks composed of HMOs, hospitals, and physicians. "We don't think that vertical integration has really worked very well in most industries," says Hutts. "We're convinced that we are going to be forming networks, so hospitals, HMOs, and physicians had better work together . . . coming together in each market." (Hutts 1995)

Owning and controlling a continuum of assets will simply not be necessary in most markets in the future. As PhyCor shows, a powerful means of delivering value is to create a vital service in a chain of services offered by a virtual network of organizations. "We want to define these virtual integration relationships and spend a lot of time on them," says Hutts. (Hutts

1995) PhyCor will hold those relationships together "by integrating with information systems, long-term contracts, sharing of managed care contracts," he adds. "All these things are going to be much more effective than actually merging your assets." (Hutts 1995)

As health care organizations struggle to define their new roles and find answers to the knotty questions of what to make and what to buy, many different business and organizational models will emerge. We believe, however, that most of them will move toward one of the following four forms (or some hybrid versions of them).

▼ *Integrated health enterprises:* A handful of enterprises like Henry Ford Health System and Allina Health System will actually do it all. Under one roof, they will offer all services to all people. We believe that such organizations will be in the minority. Although a single organization can control the entire system, rationalize resources, and manage performance, vertically integrated enterprises cost a fortune to build. They are also complex to manage and difficult to expand geographically.

▼ *Integrated delivery systems:* Many organizations, like Columbia/HCA, will combine all elements of health care delivery in a single enterprise. Such organizations will provide seamless care, offering a range of services from doctors' visits and hospital care to rehabilitation. They will actively manage system performance, rationalize resources, and collect a full stream of clinical data to improve care. Owing to their size, however, they are also complex to manage.

▼ *Health service integrators:* Some organizations, embracing virtual integration wholeheartedly, will try to manage or coordinate the entire spectrum of health services without owning any significant piece of it. Organizations such as PacifiCare and PHS, as well as many Blue Cross and Blue Shield organizations, today follow a roughly equivalent organizational model. They rely on many strong partnerships and integrate all those pieces into a seamless whole for consumers. Integrators have lots of flexibility. They can easily expand geographically, and as their ability to more comprehensively integrate information and align incentives improves, virtual integration will soon enable them to better realize substantial improvements in cost, quality, and service performance.

▼ *Niche companies:* As change continues to sweep through the industry, many new niche organizations will emerge. They will carve out specific roles, such as providing various types of care, finance and administration, purchasing, pharmaceuticals and other supplies, social services, telecommunications, media and entertainment, and information. They will deliver premium value in narrower, more specialized markets, benefiting from contracts with integrators and integrated systems. The smaller organizations will be faster moving than their larger brethren, but they will remain under heavy pressure to maintain their excellence—both in their chosen areas of competence and in building relationships.

Whichever way organizations move in the future, the most successful will be those that master the skills of managing within a virtual network. Even Allina Health System, the integrated enterprise with a 20-percent share of the Minnesota health care market, counts heavily on working within a larger virtual network. (Japsen 1994) Allina's own health plan feeds only 20 percent of the number of patients its delivery system needs to operate at capacity. As a result, Allina contracts with competing HMOs for patients to fill its hospitals, clinics, and doctors' offices. One HMO sends Allina 30 percent of its business. "There will be times you will be competing with your competitors and there will be times you will be collaborating," says chief executive Gordon Sprenger. "Competitors and collaborators may be the same parties under different circumstances." (Sprenger 1995)

## Managing Clinical Strategies

In this new world of virtual integration, the management of clinical strategies is the first essential capability that organizations need to master. That capability involves creating consistent practices across the continuum of care, including clinical practices, referral management, and case management. It also includes creating the capability to measure and improve those practices continually. The goal is for groups of virtually integrated organizations to unify medical management, delivering to consumers the best practices that yield maximum value and ever-improving health outcomes. In unified management, we believe, lies a cornerstone of competitive advantage in the future.

PacifiCare is notable among the organizations that have already grasped this new reality. Along with its four initiatives for improving service quality, the company has launched a parallel program to improve health quality. As a start, it has chosen three specific diseases to manage across the continuum: diabetes, congestive heart failure, and depression. PacifiCare believes that improving its management of those three conditions in partnership with its closest providers promises the maximum benefit for the least initial effort. "This is something that can really demonstrate our value to employers," says Ho. "Not only can we decrease group health benefits costs, but we can also increase attendance rates and productivity rates for the workforce." (Ho 1995)

As one of the first tasks of their clinical strategies effort, organizations like PacifiCare must tackle the development of clinical guidelines and care paths. Clinical guidelines provide the tools for physicians and care teams to make efficient, cost-effective, and successful clinical decisions: for example, determining when, during childbirth, a nurse needs to contact the physician and whether the physician should consider a Cesarean section. Care paths are sets of steps that provide a longitudinal focus for physicians and all other care givers who conduct and follow up on chosen treatments or procedures.

PhyCor, which manages physicians' practices as its core business, naturally puts clinical strategies at the center of its strategy. Hutts' approach has been to supply physicians with information about various clinical practices, letting the physicians convince themselves of the best clinical guidelines and care paths based on the evidence. PhyCor has created an Institute for Health Care Management where the sole intent is to identify best practice methods. Says Hutts: "What we want is to be able to share and have physicians say, 'You want it this way and I want it this other way. Isn't it interesting that you got better results than I did.... I'm going to use your method.'"(Hutts 1995)

Care paths and clinical guidelines are hardly new. A 1995 survey by Andersen Consulting shows that four out of five hospitals use care paths. (Rushing and Miller 1996) The hospitals report that paths have led to better quality, lower costs, and shorter lengths of stay. Still, most hospitals haven't taken paths very far in improving clinical practices. Most have paths for only a handful of high-volume conditions, such as bypasses and pneumonia. And although most hospitals collect variance data, only two out of three hospitals feed the data back to physicians. What's more, only one out of five runs an automated system to support care-path efforts. That means that only a tiny minority of doctors get automatic, standard variance reports. ("Clinical Path Survey" 1995) All organizations, integrated or not, need to invest in systems to identify and disseminate best practices.

Perhaps the most pointed evidence of this need was the reorganization of Allina Health System, a vertically integrated health plan and delivery organization, in early 1996. In December 1995, Sprenger announced that Allina was reorganizing its divisions around three overarching core competencies. (Sprenger 1995) One division, which would be totally integrated into the organization, would oversee the delivery of care by all hospitals and physicians. Another would manage contractual and health plan relationships. The third would manage clinical strategies, including utilization review, care path development, credentialing, and programs for health promotion. (L. Scott 1995) The goal, according to Sprenger, was to "build within the company the independence of the clinicians determining what's in the best interest of the patient." (Sprenger 1995)

To further emphasize the importance of clinical strategies, Sprenger hired a physician as the company's chief information officer. Allina's current objective is to put together an information system that supports the care givers' decision making. Sprenger says, "We cannot succeed in our integration if we cannot electronically integrate ourselves, to share best practices with our clinicians and other care givers who are spread in multiple locations all over the communities we serve." (Sprenger 1995)

As part of Allina's effort, clinical services director John Kleinman will develop models for care delivery across the continuum of care. Allina will ask that all care givers throughout its integrated delivery system apply those models. (L. Scott 1995) Such moves, says Sprenger, emanate from "a vision, a commitment to put an integrated delivery system in place that has, as its core, clinical skills." (Sprenger 1995)

That same vision must apply, with just as much urgency, to virtually integrated organizations. As at Allina, the paths will be central to the management of the continuum of care across the network of organizations in each virtual system. Winning health care enterprises will extend the scope and influence of care paths. They will create paths for many more conditions and extend those paths far beyond the hospital. The goal in each case is to assure that all physicians and care givers deliver the right services, at the right time, at the right place, in the right way. Care paths are also beginning to be extended to include consumer and employer responsibilities.

As organizations build consistent clinical strategies, along with related strategies for referral and case management, they will improve their efforts with information obtained from more effective outcomes research and management—regardless of whether they build it themselves or contract out for it. Outcomes research helps the enterprise spot emerging best practices and quickly alter guidelines, care paths, case-management procedures, wellness programs, and other policies, procedures, and practices to help consumers feel better, get well faster, and enjoy better service.

PacifiCare's health informatics department offers a straightforward illustration of the important contribution data analysis makes in improving health. As that department began collecting and analyzing hip-replacement data, it discovered that in 1994 the hip-replacement rate for the Medicare population in one physician group was close to zero. Immediately, analysts suspected that physicians in that group had been rationing care. Investigations, however, showed just the reverse. Physician assistants had visited the home of every frail, elderly patient to eliminate the hazards that could cause a fall or broken hip. In other words, the group had moved aggressively to provide preventive care and in so doing stopped the injuries from happening. (Appleby 1995) Rather than pointing to poor health care delivery, the data pointed to a simple practice for improving health.

The volume and variety of data needed for sophisticated outcomes management can seem overwhelming. Three years ago, PhyCor decided to make outcomes management a cornerstone capability and a means to differentiate itself from its competitors. PhyCor's Institute for Health Care Management now tracks three kinds of outcomes data: clinical results, functional status, and patient satisfaction. Only by tracking all three can PhyCor continually refine practices to create maximum consumer value. The effort demands a huge repository of data. Says Hutts: "Ultimately, we would like to go to a data warehouse so people can pick best practices throughout the country or within our universe." (Hutts 1995)

As health care organizations develop outcomes management to improve clinical strategies across the care continuum, they will find that their work yields important spin-off benefits. Health care purchasers who demand that providers demonstrate their competence to consumers through quantitative measures of quality care and service respond to improvements. As previously referenced, in October 1993, Kaiser Permanente publicly released a report card that divided quality into two parts: preventive care and treatment. Kaiser Permanente developed measures for effectiveness (does the organization achieve the desired health outcomes?) and appropriateness (does the organization achieve these outcomes in the most efficient manner possible?) for both preventive care and treatment. ("Measuring and Reporting" 1993)

Kaiser Permanente, for example, published data for the success of coronary artery bypass graft (CABG) surgery. Ailing heart patients can actually look up the CABG surgery mortality rate within 30 days of discharge. In 1993, it was 6.1 percent. They can also look up how it compares with a national benchmark—6.4 percent in 1993. ("Quality Report Card" 1993) As for appropriateness, Kaiser Permanente measures such parameters as the diabetes inpatient discharge rate. This measure, if unusually high, may indicate that the health plan has not been providing diabetics with the appropriate education on insulin use and self-care techniques. ("Measuring and Reporting" 1993)

Kaiser Permanente's measures include both intermediate results and outcome results. Immunization rates and prenatal care rates, for example, are intermediate measures. Outbreak rates for preventable diseases (diphtheria, tetanus) and low birthweight rates are outcomes measures. ("Measuring and Reporting" 1993) The combination of so many measures yields a complete picture of Kaiser Permanente's quality of service and care. Those measures become an effective means for Kaiser Permanente to differentiate itself from competitors to win employers' business.

Although organizations like Kaiser Permanente have already taken huge strides in measuring outcomes, their progress to date will almost certainly pale in comparison to what lies in the future. Most organizations capture and use only a small fraction of available data. Those that rapidly upgrade their ability to monitor their performance, measure gaps, and take steps to improve will build much stronger clinical management capabilities than their competitors. Additionally, the organizations that reveal their measures publicly may soon begin winning more business than others that lack that prowess in outcomes management. Today's vertically integrated organizations generally lead the health industry in outcomes management, but virtually integrated organizations have the potential to use information technology to build and enhance this expertise quickly. In every case, what counts most is a strong capability to measure the value delivered to consumers across the continuum of care.

### Optimizing Supply and Demand

The second essential capability for organizations to manage within integrated, virtual organizations is optimizing supply and demand. This means managing the demand for care and in turn the supply of care so that the two roughly match. Today they rarely do. Patients too often pile up in waiting rooms, as their demand overwhelms the supply of care givers. Or, conversely, health care staff sit around idly as nobody shows up to call on their services. At the moment, few organizations skillfully optimize demand and supply to match consumer needs. In the future, however, all organizations must.

Simultaneously, organizations must also apply incentives that encourage consumers to use only appropriate care across the continuum. Organizations will have to experiment with higher copayments for care, bonuses for preventive care, premium discounts for healthy lifestyles, and medical savings accounts that encourage thrift in using services.

While organizations struggle to reduce demand for unnecessary care, they must also manage supply. Few organizations, virtually integrated or not, skillfully and efficiently manage their resources—staff, equipment, and facilities—to meet demand. Today, supply and demand rarely match. Consumers complain of spending two, four, or six hours of time away from work or home to get ten minutes of attention from a care professional. Meanwhile, hospitals, clinics, and physician practices worry about overspending on staff and facilities, sending their costs way beyond those of their competitors.

Today, organizations face an exciting opportunity to improve the balance of supply and demand. They already accumulate data, in hospital records, appointment books, and demographic profiles, that project future demand. They must now develop the systems to forecast and respond to day-to-day, week-to-week, and month-to-month demand. Although many organizations use data to adjust supply over the very long term (a year or more), or the very short term (within several hours of a shift change), they can do much better. They must develop the capability to feed data into new, more sophisticated systems for forecasting, master scheduling, and managing the utilization of staff, facilities, and equipment.

By analyzing their data in combination with farsighted tools such as life care plans, winning organizations will find that demand forecasting is not as difficult as it might seem. Analysis of emergency room data, use of community health services, volumes of outpatient visits, and so on will show that past demand patterns roughly resemble future patterns. For example, seasonal influenza in the frail elderly is a relatively predictable event. Based on international epidemiological data, it is possible to predict the virus type and estimate its impact on this fragile, older population. With this information the health care organization can implement prevention around an aggressive vaccination policy to protect as many people as possible. Concurrently, the organization can use the data to insure that the appropriate providers and facilities accommodate the demands of this population. Because of the special nursing needs of the severely ill elderly, a focused approach can make a significant difference in the quality and cost-effectiveness of their care.

Managing resources requires that organizations develop better macro- and microforecasting skills. By macroforecasting, we mean the ability to forecast overall demand for services within a hospital, health plan, or network of providers. Macroforecasting enables organizations to size and configure the overall delivery network, as well as allocate staff and services to meet demand at the individual facility level. By microforecasting, we mean the ability to forecast care demand hour by hour in clinics, physician practices, emergency rooms, hospitals, and other facilities a few days or weeks ahead of time. Together, macro- and microforecasting enable enterprises to align supply and demand and to respond more quickly to consumer demands for care.

In physician group practices, for example, clerks can continually recalculate expected demand up to four weeks into the future. With scheduling software that can show daily peaks and valleys of expected demand, staff can juggle appointments to coincide with capacity. Such forecasting cannot eliminate unexpected surges in demand, but it can level the fluctuations so common in practices that ignore data hidden in years of appointment books.

The ultimate goal of some virtually integrated organizations is to develop supply and demand management capabilities that are strong enough to support a closed-loop resource management system. Such integration allows organizations to merge data from outcomes systems, care path systems, and supply management systems. The outcomes-management system continually feeds back data to improve care paths. The care paths continually feed back data to improve management of supply. Both the care path and demand-management systems feed back results data to the outcomes system. A closed-loop system can leverage all the information collected in every aspect of health care and service across the continuum of care. The closed-loop resource management system gives the virtual organization an unbeatable advantage over other organizations. Few organizations have progressed very far in the creation of such systems, but the winners in health care will be those organizations that do create them—and use them.

Some organizations propose to eventually connect their life care plans to demand forecasts. The life care plans, connected to longitudinal care paths, will calculate demand for certain categories of care, giving plans and providers a macro view of demands as much as a year into the future, along with a micro view into the demands of individual patients anywhere from a day to a month in advance. Taken to the limit, these systems would be able to forecast demand for preventive, chronic, acute, and elective care for scores of conditions and generate a schedule of demands for staff, equipment, and facilities.

### Managing Relationships

Many organizations have long considered relationship management as merely a nicety: a good idea nobody ever gets to. In managing the virtual organization, however, building strong, enduring relationships is a third critical capability. Three kinds of relationships remain primary: those with purchasers, providers, and suppliers. Some organizations will form virtual links with all three, as well as with a variety of other health care players. The goal is to string together the employers, government agencies, drug makers, medical device manufacturers, physicians, health plans, hospitals, rehab facilities, and other organizations into one smoothly coordinated whole. Mutual success is the result of a partnership strategy and structure through which the entire virtual organization delivers the maximum value to consumers across the continuum of health care.

Once again, PacifiCare is a good example of a company leading the way in virtual integration across the continuum. The company has even suggested breaking the industry standard one-year purchaser health plan contract. PacifiCare's

Sam Ho wants to encourage purchasers to cut five-year contracts. (Ho 1995) The longer period, he says, will allow PacifiCare to realize a return on its long-term investments in improving the quality and efficiency of care. It would also enhance PacifiCare's accountability, giving it enough time to accumulate data that demonstrates improved outcomes to employers.

Like Ho, we believe a virtual system that includes the health plan, providers, employers, and individual consumers will yield significantly better outcomes than the traditional arm's-length contracting approach. This thinking marks a sea change for health plans, but it promises employers and consumers lower health care premiums, fewer lost work days, and higher productivity.

The formula that makes each partnership endure will vary. But we believe that health care enterprises face two main challenges: to align incentives and share information. Information sharing poses huge technical and cultural challenges. It requires many organizations to exchange data rapidly and routinely—data on everything from benefits and administration to clinical practices, demand optimization, and resource management. Aligning incentives requires partners to craft trusting relationships that encourage participants to make each other winners. As Joe Hutts of PhyCor says, "If you are in business with somebody—particularly in partnerships—strategic strengths are important, capital strengths are important, managed care skills are important. But if they know that they can trust you and you have their best interest at heart, that is most powerful of all." (Hutts 1995)

### Aligning Incentives

One organization that has built scores of partnerships on the basis of shared incentives is Physicians Health Services (PHS), the Connecticut-based company known to its admirers as the physician-friendly HMO. PHS got its start by organizing Connecticut physicians into independent physician associations, or IPAs, and contracting with them for services. (Natt 1995) From the beginning, PHS's structure gave physicians tremendous influence. To this day, a number of physicians sit on PHS's board, and physicians can vote on a variety of issues.

More recently, PHS has embarked on an expansion into New York and New Jersey. The speed of that expansion has demanded that PHS rely heavily on its skill in crafting win/win partnerships. The most visible of recent partnerships, one that best illustrates the art of aligning incentives, is the alliance of PHS with Guardian Life, one of the nation's largest indemnity insurers.

The alliance between the HMO and the traditional insurer evolved as a result of executives in each company searching for a way to overcome the most pressing challenges in their respective businesses. PHS, facing rapid industry consolidation, had to grow rapidly; otherwise it would be the acquisition prey of a larger competitor. Executives were convinced that they had only 18 months to establish a position in the New York market before competitors would gain impregnable market share and market power. PHS launched its expansion plans, signing up physicians in New York and on Long Island with the knowledge that it was gambling a huge amount of investors' cash and patience on less than surefire plans. (Elrod 1995) Executives feared that PHS might not grow fast enough.

Guardian Life faced an even greater challenge. It was confronted with aggressive HMO marketing strategies and unique product designs in the New York area. Employers and employees were being lured into managed care with premiums that were one-third of the cost of medical indemnity premiums. Guardian had no comparable product for its clients but was committed to retaining its position in the health insurance market. The solution—search for a partner to achieve this goal.

"We didn't want to compromise our position as a quality provider of medical benefits," says Jack Pallotta, senior vice president of Guardian Life and architect of the ultimate deal with Paul Philpott, senior vice president at PHS. "Our concerns were that we did not have a cultural understanding and technical expertise to take control of a managed care product. Since speed to market was the most critical factor, it wasn't feasible to develop the necessary databases, physician relationships, advertising campaigns, and pricing methodologies in-house." (Pallotta 1995)

Guardian and PHS came to recognize that a deal would be successful only if the strategic interests of both organizations were satisfied within the partnership. PHS saw that by leveraging Guardian's more than 1,000 New York area brokers it could amass market share rapidly and penetrate the small-business market. Guardian saw that by offering a managed care health plan under the name of a physician-friendly HMO, it would be able to retain customers (and profit) from sales that the company would otherwise lose to managed care competitors.

Once the companies signed the joint venture deal, they benefited immediately. PHS was able to gain incredible momentum in the New York market. In the first nine months of the Guardian-PHS joint venture, approximately 50,000 New Yorkers signed up for PHS's product. The alliance was the key that unlocked the success of PHS's strategy. "One way we would fail in New York is to take too long to get up and going—too long to develop that delivery system, too long to get a brokerage relationship, too long to get our own sales people really pumped up," says PHS chief executive Mickey Herbert.

"In the history of this company written 30 years from now, I think that may be the biggest determinant of our success in New York: We were able to unleash 1,000 brokers into this market." (Herbert 1995)

Guardian and PHS grasped from the start the power of aligning incentives. Their deal specifies profit sharing as equal partners. Says PHS's Philpott: "Our future is totally dependent on our mutual success." (Philpott 1995)

If in a group with 100 employees, ninety-nine bought Guardian's indemnity insurance and only one bought PHS's HMO product, Guardian and PHS would split the profits evenly. If ninety-nine bought PHS's product and only one bought Guardian's, the two would still share profits evenly. Guardian began the joint venture with a much larger New York customer base, but it gambled that it would ultimately make more money in a venture selling both HMO and indemnity products than relying on its declining indemnity business. (Philpott 1995; Elrod 1995; Pallotta 1995)

Another company that has built its business on the innovative partnerships that reflect win/win incentives is Columbia/HCA, the nation's largest hospital chain. In June 1994, for example, Columbia announced a joint venture with Southwest Texas Methodist Hospital in San Antonio. By merging Columbia's four San Antonio hospitals and two surgery centers with Methodist, Columbia was able to assemble the Methodist Healthcare System of San Antonio. The system comprises five hospitals with 1,500 beds, two outpatient surgery centers, and a full continuum of services ranging from complex organ transplants and neurosurgery to psychiatric care and home health services. For Columbia, the deal yielded a bigger, more comprehensive and more profitable delivery system. By installing new information systems and taking advantage of Columbia's purchasing power, the joint venture saved $5 million its first year alone.

The partnership operates according to the Social Principles of the United Methodist Church. Methodist's share of profits from the joint venture will fund such community outreach services as child immunization programs, health education programs, and inner-city health clinics. The result is that while cutting care costs, the joint venture expands its availability, especially to San Antonio's poor. (Columbia/HCA Annual Report 1994)

Yet another company that has built its business on win/win partnerships is Baxter Healthcare. In fact, one of Baxter's more recent deals is with the new Methodist Healthcare System. In late 1995, after the Columbia/HCA agreement, Methodist called Baxter, asking executives to examine the possibility of expanding its just-in-time supply arrangement into a far-reaching program for managing and cutting costs across Methodist's entire system of hospitals and outpatient centers. ("Baxter, Columbia" 1996) Methodist called for Baxter's virtual integration of its entire menu of hospital management services with Methodist's hospital operations. Baxter would become one of Methodist's key operational managers.

In an example of true virtual integration, Baxter has since taken on a broad range of system functions, including supply replenishment, in-hospital distribution, sterile processing, laundry and linen management, surgical-supply kitting, and clinical process standardization. Baxter has also placed a full-time consultant, a former operating room nurse, at Methodist to work with physicians and nurses on a daily basis to establish clinical-care strategies based on Baxter's "best demonstrated" practices database. By bringing its distribution, logistics, and clinical consulting expertise to bear, Baxter estimates it will help save Methodist more than $60 million over the course of five years while generating $115 million in revenue for Baxter. (Graham 1995; "Baxter, Columbia" 1996)

The most remarkable aspect of the deal, however, is the incentive agreement. Baxter's cost-management spin-off, Allegiance Healthcare, will earn a fee for its services and will share evenly with the Methodist Healthcare System any cost savings or increases that stem from its consulting and management work. In other words, Baxter will share in both the gains and losses that result from its recommendations.

We believe similar gain-sharing agreements will become standard practice in virtual organizations. The age-old practice of allying with a partner as a preliminary to acquiring it will not pay off for companies seeking to supplement their repertoire of core competencies; such short-sighted vision will lead instead to conflict, lost opportunities, and partnership failure. The crafting of agreements that spread the risks among all parties will prevail. To date, in fact, Baxter has signed seventeen agreements in which each partner shares the risks and rewards equally. ("Baxter, Columbia" 1996)

Given that physicians occupy a primary role in controlling health care cost and quality, innovative incentive structures must extend to physicians and physician practices. When Columbia/HCA takes over the operation of a hospital, for example, it often sells the doctors a small stake in the facility. Critics charge that the practice is a conflict of interest for physicians, who can better line their pocketbooks by shunting charity cases to other hospitals. All the same, the practice does awaken in physicians a keener understanding of the economics of running a hospital. (Schiller et al. 1995: 80)

Many health care organizations have their physician incentives backwards. PhyCor's Hutts notes that many managed care organizations are wrong to put independent physicians on salary. "It occurred to us early on that this had problems," he says. "Every company I have ever been a part of was always trying to get the employees to think and act like owners, whereas here we have a whole industry in which we're making owners into employees." (Hutts 1995)

PhyCor buys the assets of physician practices, pays the physicians about 40 percent in PhyCor stock, and shares subsequent profits of the practice with them. "Our whole thrust has been to keep physicians in ownership," says Hutts. "We negotiate a 40-year agreement, we have parallel incentives, we both have an interest in the company. If they get hurt, we get hurt. If we do well, they do well. The whole thing revolves around them continuing to be owners with a business partner. That has been very powerful." (Hutts 1995)

### Sharing Information

The second challenge in building virtual organizations is sharing information. Information sharing fuels the search for creative solutions that yield increasingly competitive efficiencies, quality, and service. On the one hand, this means creating a cultural attitude that gets people to disseminate their insights, fresh ideas, and performance data—both good news and bad. On the other, it means setting up systems to transmit easily all necessary administrative and clinical data among the partnering organizations. For example, providers must set themselves up to transmit admissions, discharges, referral requests, authorization requests, eligibility and benefit inquiries, and clinical data to health plans. Health plans, in turn, have to transmit similar data to providers: case management notes, remittances, claims inquiry responses, and so on. Additionally, succeeding at more advanced stages of medical management will require much more extensive sharing of medical and clinical information among the various entities in a virtual organization, including the end consumer, who must also be a part of this virtual value chain. Such communication requires sophisticated information systems and, ultimately, the Health Information Infocosm, which we discuss further in Chapter 12.

As organizations share information, one of the most important skills to build is continual feedback among partners, particularly when that feedback contributes to a closed-loop resource management system. Virtually integrated health systems need to capitalize at every turn on their knowledge, becoming every bit as much a learning organization as each enterprise within the system. The same principles of information capture, analysis, and dissemination discussed earlier in this chapter and in other chapters apply across the virtual organization. When Columbia measures the outcomes from among its many facilities, for example, it continually feeds the performance data back to the doctors at hundreds of different hospitals around the United States. "We try to measure as many outcomes as we can, and then we share ideas," says president and CEO Rick Scott. "We don't believe that sitting in our Nashville headquarters office we know how you should change in McMinnville, Tennessee. But we know that through measurement, we can show how someone else is practicing differently and getting better outcomes. That will ensure change." (R. Scott 1995)

Making that happen, of course, requires more than simple sharing. We believe that virtual organizations must establish teams both within and across enterprises to interpret and act on the information they receive. Multifunctional teams dedicated to building relationships with purchasers would benefit from complete information on the needs of each employer's population of employees as well as detailed information on each employee. With that information, teams from marketing, sales, and other functions would work with purchasers to design tailored health plans. A purchaser worried about too many on-the-job injuries, for example, would submit information that might suggest services stressing health and safety education, preventive exercise regimes, and self-care for such ailments as lower back pain.

Because teams would work with purchasers, providers, and health plans throughout the processes of enrollment, service delivery, claims, and customer service, they would obtain huge amounts of information from their partners, much in the same way as Baxter had to obtain detailed cost and utilization data before its virtual integration with Methodist Healthcare System. Only with that information could the teams tackle such tasks as installing paperless transaction-processing systems among virtual partners or standardizing clinical practices among providers of the virtual organization.

We stress the importance of information and incentives to the success of managing the virtual organization. They are critical and too often neglected. We do not believe, however, that shared incentives and information will alone guarantee the success of partnerships and virtual integration. Many other factors figure into success: strategic fit, mutual trust, alignment of values, sharing power, streamlining processes, complementary competencies, and clear governance structures. But winning health care organizations must not overlook the sticky issues that can otherwise cause virtual integration to founder.

Ultimately, the goal of the virtual organization is to create an enormously complex, tightly interconnected system. Many of the required skills draw managers into unfamiliar territory, calling on them to coordinate as never before. Virtual management and especially the capabilities of clinical strategies management, supply and demand optimization, and relationship management will determine which organizations (in the language of PacifiCare) most quickly find winning solutions to the value equation.

# REFERENCES

Appleby, Chuck. 1995. The measure of medical services. *Hospitals & Health Networks,* June 20, 26–28, 30, 32, 34.

Baxter, Columbia sign agreement for first-of-its kind program to reduce health care costs. 1996. PRNewswire.

Clinical path survey: a study of clinical path trends in health care. August 1995. Unpublished report. Andersen Consulting.

Columbia/HCA Annual Report. 1994. Nashville: Columbia/HCA.

Elrod, Jim. 1995. Interview with Ken Jennings and Sharyn Materna.

Graham, Jennifer. 1995. Interview with Ken Jennings and Jay Saddler. Deerfield, Ill.

Herbert, Mickey. 1995. Interview with Ken Jennings, Wendy Kingsbury, and Ian Galliot. October 17.

Ho, Sam. 1995. Interview with Kurt Miller and Bill Combs. Pittsburgh, Penn.

Hutts, Joe. 1995. Interview with David Osborne and Mike Raney.

Japsen, Bruce. 1994. Allina deal shows market trends. *Modern Healthcare,* August 8, 56.

Kroll, E. E., et al. 1995. PacifiCare: company report. Lehman Brothers, Inc., March 29.

Manley, Mike. 1995. Interview with Erik Hansen. December 22.

Measuring and reporting healthcare quality. 1993. Unpublished report. Andersen Consulting.

Natt, Bob. 1995. Interview with Ken Jennings.

Olmos, David R. 1994. PacifiCare offers new medical plan for large firms. *Los Angeles Times,* November 2, D1.

Pallotta, Jack. 1995. Interview with Ken Jennings.

Philpott, Paul. 1995. Interview with Ken Jennings, Sharyn Materna, and Wendy Kingsbury.

Quality Report Card. 1993. Unpublished report. Kaiser Permanente Northern California Region.

Rushing, Steve, and Kurt Miller. 1996. New survey reveals growing importance of clinical paths. Healthcare marketing memo, January 17.

Schiller, Zachary, et al. 1995. Balance sheets that get well soon. *Business Week*, September 4, 80–81, 84.

Scott, Lisa. 1995. Allina redraws operating divisions. *Modern Healthcare*, December 18–25.

Scott, Rick. 1995. Interview with Ken Jennings. September 6.

Sprenger, Gordon. 1995. Interview with Ken Jennings and Rich Moore.

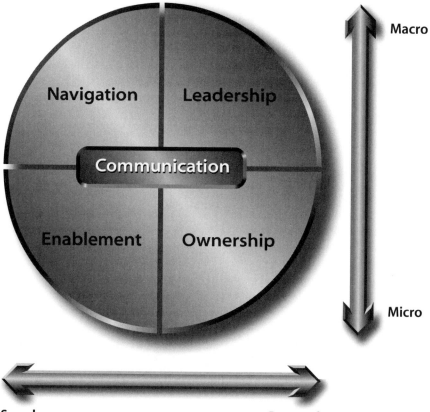

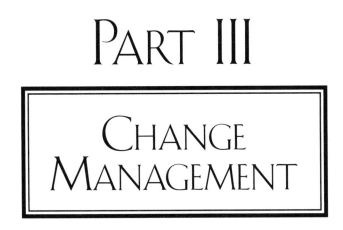

# PART III

## CHANGE MANAGEMENT

A s much as half of a health care organization's operating costs stem from hiring, training, compensating, and supporting employees. No wonder, then, that so many executives say that people are their most important asset. And no wonder that the return on the people investment can dictate whether an organization will win or lose. A low or declining return will relegate an organization to the dustbin of competitiveness.

That is why one of the biggest challenges for health care organizations in the future is change or, more accurately, the handling of the management of change. Too often managers trying to transform their organizations drive people to the water cooler, where employees wring their hands over job losses, commiserate over low morale, and snipe at unclear mission statements. The result: People's productivity and morale plunge. No amount of clarity in strategy, as discussed in Part I, or level of competency, as covered in Part II, will resuscitate the flagging fortunes of an organization caught in such a malaise.

We offer the means for overcoming this malaise: a full-scale program of change management. That is the subject of the third part of our book, which concludes our exploration of the three essential phases in transforming health care organizations to winning enterprises of the future: creating strategy, building competencies, and managing change.

Change management is a discipline that assures that organizations and employees meet new and existing performance targets rapidly and effectively. It prescribes the creation or refinement of new management practices and processes, organization structures, culture, and competencies for superior human performance. Without change management, employee thumb twiddling, furtive job hunting, foot dragging, and just plain fretting will stymie an organization's progress toward the sought-after goal of market leadership.

The practice of change management builds on two assumptions. The first is that people's performance, the time they spend applying their energies versus airing their anxieties, directly impacts business performance. Change managers need to figure out what aspects of human performance must change to enable the organization to meet business objectives. The second assumption is that an organization can devise an approach to preserve revenues, profits, lean cost structures, share prices, or other financial objectives even during the upheaval of a change program. Management must adopt those techniques that can help an organization jump to a new and better future without slipping en route into the financial pits.

Although every organization will travel a different "change journey," depending on the drivers and scope of change, every well-managed change program will deliver four enticing benefits:

▼ *Faster change:* Employees meet performance targets on time and on budget. The faster people meet their targets, the more value the organization can deliver to consumers.

▼ *More loyal stakeholders:* Loyal consumers, employees, suppliers, shareholders, and other stakeholders help the organization continually boost revenue, ally with strong business partners, obtain equity and debt capital, and attract talented new employees.

▼ *Lower risks:* The change program will proceed with lower risks—of quality lapses, budgetary crises, hostile takeover suitors, and failed initiatives to develop new businesses.

▼ *Higher capacity for future change:* The workforce will develop an enduring new competency—the ability to change quickly. A high change capacity enables the organization to set higher change goals and meet them more rapidly in the future.

The next four chapters show how the feat of changing while delivering such benefits is possible. Chapter by chapter we examine the four requirements for successful transformation: creating the best leaders, inspiring a real sense of ownership, enabling the change to occur smoothly by aligning policies with people's skills and talents, and navigating through the barriers that stand in the way of progress.

Leadership, ownership, enablement, navigation—mastering these four components of change management will help health care managers deliver solid results as they transform themselves to winning health care enterprises of the future.

Organizations that do not use change-management techniques will suffer in a purgatory of mediocrity. They will fail to reach targets on time, waste resources fighting avoidable conflict between stakeholders, and undercut employee and investor confidence in management. They will bring down on their heads not just a reputation for lousy performance but impotence in pursuing agendas for future change and improvement.

As Sumantra Ghoshal of the London Business School says, "The role of management must change . . . from structuring tasks to shaping behavior." Managers who don't grasp this new reality will saddle their organizations with an intolerable handicap. This third part of our book explains how to avoid that handicap and, more important, turn change management into a personal and organizational strength.

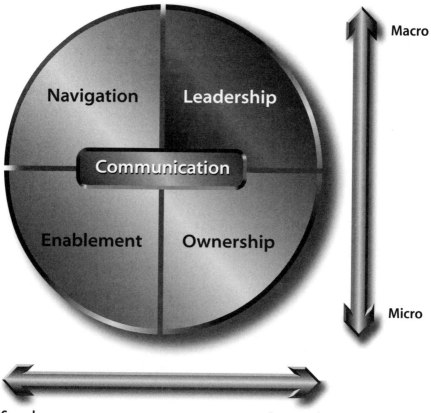

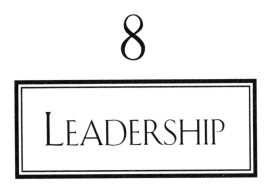

# 8

# LEADERSHIP

Poised like a sentry at the door of corporate headquarters of Aetna Health Plans, the 1958 Cadillac Fleetwood drew sighs of admiration for yesterday's fine fins, massive motor, and wide whitewalls. Its huge chrome bumpers caught fire from the sun, and its black surface gleamed, despite minor scratches from four decades of use. Next to it, a sleek silver Infiniti offered a stark contrast in modern art and technology: speed and power and style shimmering in readiness. Parked at a slight angle to each other so that everyone entering the building had to pass between them, the two cars caused a stir of curiosity and puzzlement among employees.

Once inside, they gathered with executives to discuss the future of the health care organization and the changes that Aetna would need to make to stay competitive. Jamie McClain, the former CEO, began with an analogy: "Like the Cadillac, we were the best," he told the troops, "tops in the field. All the competition wanted to imitate us. Today's marketplace, however, is a new course. There are just too many fast cars on the market, and we can't keep driving the same old car, no matter how good it's been for us. We're heading into uncharted territory, and we're in for the ride of our lives. That's why I parked an Infiniti out there. We've got to be better than good. We've got to define the new standard for the best!"

Corporations are learning today that they cannot run well just by changing the spark plugs. Even an old-fashioned overhaul won't get you onto the expressway faster—not if your enterprise is still armored in steel. Chugging along as the avatar of inefficiency, the old organization just can't keep pace on the speedways of today's health care industry.

The next four chapters analyze what drives that execution, what the transformed enterprise needs to do to translate strategies and competencies into action. Any change, of course, disrupts old behaviors and expectations. No matter how positive, change threatens us with the feeling that we are no longer in control. We, in short, are used to old accelerators.

Operating at full-throttle takes the sure hand of a practiced driver. In this chapter we begin an analysis of change management by introducing some of the most effective leaders we have met in the health care industry. Each has a distinctive driving style; each takes the direction that he or she believes is best for the organization: Some race along new courses, while others seek well-traveled routes to their destinations. All, however, are dedicated to the transformation journey, and they are all demonstrably outstanding leaders in the health care industry.

What follows a leader defines him or her: people, venture capital, a battalion of soldiers, or lemmings in a mass migration to the precipice. Leaders are there to point the direction, set the agenda, make the decisions. They need not be visionaries, but they must always inspire others to see with their clarity. They need not be authority figures, but they must always speak with authority. They need not delegate responsibility, but they must always be responsible for their delegations.

Many industries have for years suffered from a lack of good leadership. And, perhaps, no industry has suffered that lack more than health care, which, according to its most knowledgeable critics, has been underled and overmanaged. One CEO of a major health plan, for example, refers to the Taj Mahals of the health care industry where managers don't understand the product they are managing. He points a critical finger at the industry for maintaining the illusion that it needed only to find competent managers who would wrap the hospital, the clinic, the pharmaceutical company, or the HMO in the mantle of "business as usual."

Today's large health care organizations are complex amalgams of independent clinicians, administrative personnel, shareholders, and even other organizations. Accordingly, their leaders must manage a complex set of constituents and partners. Given those requirements, it is no wonder that an effective leader is a precious commodity.

We are fortunate to have discovered a wealth of great leaders. In our conversations with executives throughout the health care industry, we had many opportunities to observe leaders who are directing their health care enterprises through major change projects. Each organization has set as goals some of the strategies we outlined in earlier chapters to position itself at the head of the market.

We observed that leaders conducted the key change projects in three stages: planning and launching the transformation, executing the plan, and sustaining the changes. If it were merely following those three activities in sequence, we might offer a general map that any would-be skipper could take to the bridge. We have learned from our interviews with industry leaders, however, that rarely is the change process so linear. Their stories testify to the need for iterative management and the flexibility to meet new challenges as they arise. Whether directing the course of a huge health care enterprise or a small start-up business, no sooner does one launch a change program than a new wind blows up to push the organization off course. Responding with a sure hand and a practiced eye will help ensure that the ship stays in the channel.

In our interviews, executives confirm that their health care enterprises must realistically evaluate their strategies, competencies, and the market conditions that drive change. In tailoring a change program, there is no one-size-fits-all garment. Although each enterprise must fashion its own response, we believe that we can learn general lessons by studying the models those leaders have established.

### *Planning and Launching the Transformation*

Leaders are well acquainted with fire. Sometimes it is a match held to their feet: Profits drop for several successive quarters, an acquisition fails, enrollments in health plans continue on a downward spiral. Sometimes, however, the heat emanates from a corporate meltdown.

When the heat is on, some organizations look outside for a savior who can bring fresh insights, valuable experience, and the knowledge of other transformations to direct the current project.

Consider the case of St. Vincent's Hospital, a 480-bed teaching and tertiary-care facility in Melbourne (Victoria State), Australia. Founded by the Sisters of Charity in 1893, the hospital's strong sense of values focused on health care for people who could least afford it; accordingly, executives had

had to make sacrifices in caring for the physical plant and administering many of the hospital's processes. Although St. Vincent's had earned respect for its core specialties in cardiology and heart surgery, it could no longer keep pace with fierce competitors. Its technology was out of date, and its public funding had declined severely; the corporate culture was firmly entrenched and resistant to change.

Enter Dr. David Campbell, who became CEO in 1992. His appointment as senior executive marked a clear departure from the conservative direction the hospital had taken over its 100-year history. Both a medical doctor and a professional hospital administrator, Campbell recognized the danger signs and set about to rescue the hospital from sure collapse. His ability to help St. Vincent's change from the status of an old Cadillac to that of a new Infiniti exemplifies the kind of leadership that we believe is essential for the successful transformation of today's health care enterprises. Leaders must set the direction for the transformation, prioritizing initiatives, articulating the need for change, and enlisting everyone's support. They must create an atmosphere conducive to change (Reinertsen 1994), injecting a sense of dissatisfaction with the status quo and energizing everyone to undertake the transformation.

### Setting Direction: How to Leave a Burning Platform

Campbell's arrival at St. Vincent's Hospital was none too soon. To appropriate a metaphor suggested by Darryl Conner in his recent book *Managing at the Speed of Change* (1992), we would say that the organization was standing on a "burning platform." The prospect of jumping into the North Sea below is not very appealing, but the alternative is a lot worse. Campbell recalls the daunting set of crisis-level problems that greeted his arrival: The hospital's hundred-year-old infrastructure stood in need of major repairs, and the staff worked with inadequate computer systems and did not have the technological training to enter the information age. In short, St. Vincent's could not satisfy the health care requirements of the community it served. "We were trying to move from the nineteenth century to the twenty-first century in one go," Campbell says. (Campbell 1995) Today, a little more than two years into the transformation, the enterprise is adding sophisticated information technology and showing how it can participate in the global health care network.

Campbell tells the story of one executive who, at a meeting of St. Vincent's senior hospital staff, wrote out a cryptic equation: "SVH = B(3V5A 10/10W)." When staff members expressed their bewilderment, the executive translated for them: "St. Vincent's Hospital will be the best in three years in Victoria, in five years in Australia, and in 10 years one of the 10 best hospitals in the world." Although skeptics dismissed the formula as a pipe dream, it appeared on St. Vincent's vision document, and it became the motto that has energized everyone—hospital staff and customers—in imagining a transformed St. Vincent's. Everyone embraced the hospital's commitment to meeting, exceeding, and in some cases actually setting the standards for best practices. ("Understanding Enterprise Transformation" 1995)

## Creating Dissatisfaction with the Status Quo

The St. Vincent's formula is a splendid example of how leaders launch a substantial change program by creating a sense that the organization can no longer afford to conduct business as usual. David Campbell reports that St. Vincent's invited 400 senior staff members—including doctors, nurses, and other clinicians—to a two-day course where they learned to stretch their managerial muscles, as well as their understanding of the changes that lie before the entire industry. "People at St. Vincent's," Campbell says, "need to understand the big picture and the forces that are shaping the global health system as well as the ones that are forcing change at the level of the organization." That confrontation with people from various areas of the hospital has had its painful moments: Physicians challenged administrators about industry standards for care, nurses disagreed with physicians over what constitutes speedy outcomes, and administrators tried to impress on staff members the reality of market forces.

One of the best ways to create dissatisfaction with the status quo is to demonstrate the kind of progress others have made in their transformations. Capitalizing on the natural tendency to compare, a number of executives these days lead their own seminars: They invite corporate officials from within their organizations or from rival institutions to convene, offer testimonials, and practice the fine art of collaborative thinking. PhyCor, for instance, under the direction of CEO Joe Hutts, now offers a key leadership institute several times a year. Presidents of clinics, executive directors, medical personnel, and directors of managed care groups gather to discuss strategies, seek resolutions of common problems, and assess the new performance standards for the industry as a whole. When people cannot attend the seminars, PhyCor sends teams of experts to them. These experts have proven records of successfully managing clinics and attacking problems head-on. They are eager to work with staff and management at other clinics who are just beginning to institute major change programs of their own. At its Camp Caduceus, PhyCor's medical directors from specific regions of the country discuss technical procedures and plot the most effective use of their knowledge and experience. (Hutts 1995)

## Articulating the Need for Change

If you're planning to launch a major change in your organization, you must articulate it clearly for everyone, not just the members of the executive team. As experienced CEOs told us, their success was due, in large part, to their willingness to talk frankly to people throughout their organizations. Those executives often refer to going out into "the field" and talking to "the troops."

Tom Peters (1987) calls that technique "management by wandering around," and it is one that Gordon Sprenger at Allina Health System has made into a hallmark of his leadership style. Despite Allina's massive size—18 hospitals, 64 physicians' clinics, more than 400 physicians, and 20,000 employees—Sprenger pays regular visits, even to groups that are farthest from the organization's headquarters in Minnetonka, Minnesota.

While this is certainly not breakthrough thinking, it is a significant challenge for leaders to make the commitment in time and energy necessary to do it well.

For all the lip service they pay to creating a productive corporate culture, many CEOs prefer to remain holed up in their executive suites, where they are least effective when it comes to managing a change program. When they are out of the trenches, they lose the opportunity to talk directly with employees, to clarify for them the goals of the change program and help allay their fears and concerns. Great leaders not only leave their doors open but also visit with the people down the hall and across the stockroom floor.

Terry White, the CEO of MetroHealth, for example, believes in bringing everyone into the program for change. Accordingly, he invited all 3,000 Metro employees to attend question and answer forums, and he rarely passed up an opportunity for a one-on-one discussion in the hallway or the cafeteria. Describing himself as the leader of a leadership team, a group of some of the most inventive people at Metro-Health, White guides the company's change management program—or, to be more exact, he allows the team to do the guiding. At their Tuesday afternoon meetings, for example, team members participate in roundtable discussions, reporting to the group rather than to White. He prefers the role of facilitator, helping to build a sense of community by giving people the chance to present their ideas.

### Creating an Atmosphere for Change

As Terry White and other corporate leaders have learned, such meetings force the oil-and-water mixture of attitudes and assumptions about both the organization and the direction that the entire industry is taking. This is exactly what will make leaders set a new strategy for the health care industry. No one comes away from such meetings without some sense of dissatisfaction about health care and its future.

Dr. Ronald Heifitz, a surgeon and psychiatrist who directs the Leadership Education Project at Harvard's Kennedy School of Government, believes that disorientation is valuable in helping people to make changes, so long as they do not experience overwhelming and debilitating distress. (Flower 1995: 32) Although people are likely, at first, to resist the transformation, a good leader can help them see that failure to change will eventually create more pain than they now fear. The great leaders know precisely how much pressure to create at this early stage of the transformation: Too much dissatisfaction will drive the best people away, too little and people won't give the program serious consideration.

Our interviews with health care executives suggest that there are three main elements that create dissatisfaction with the status quo: first, building and developing a compelling vision of where the organization needs to go and what it needs to become; second, creating enough pain that people are willing to abandon the status quo, even if it has seemed safe up until this point; and third, making both the vision and the pain personal and immediate rather than abstract and distant.

## *Developing a Compelling Vision for the Change Initiative*

By executing a well-known technique, Joe Hutts, the CEO of PhyCor, which has seen rapid growth in the last few years, recommends articulating the company's strategic vision and key values clearly and succinctly. PhyCor, in fact, puts it all on a single sheet of paper. Everybody gets a copy, and everybody has a sense of participating in the company's future growth. Hutts sees a major challenge in the effort to establish values clearly and use these to form trusting relationships with HMOs, hospitals, and physicians. (Hutts 1995)

As people throughout the organization get a better sense of what ails it or where it is vulnerable to the forces of change, its leaders need to transform that dissatisfaction into a commitment to the change initiative. That is not work for a magician or a leadership guru. As David Campbell puts it, an effective leader has to demonstrate a range of skills in communication, coordination, strategy, and negotiation. (Campbell 1995) St. Vincent's offered particular challenges in that regard: Its people were deeply committed to the religious values that informed the hospital's philosophy. A major aspect of that change program, therefore, involved convincing everyone that without abandoning their values, they could think in more secular terms about their service to the community. They had to think about how they could best deliver health care in an uncertain world.

People's attitudes are tight springs that must be wound even tighter before they can be released. Too much stress can suddenly snap the spring, but successful leaders apply just the right pressure to accomplish the release. Frank communication has always been the best tool for prying loose the most tightly held beliefs. At St. Vincent's, for example, Campbell had tables set up in the Bistro every Wednesday for six weeks so employees could respond to the change initiatives, make suggestions for improvements, and participate in the issues under debate.

When people can voice their ideas in a forum, they are much more likely to adopt the effort on a personal level and devote their energies to seeing the initiative to its conclusion. The effective leader seeks to enhance such an atmosphere, even though not everyone in the organization will be completely enthusiastic about all the changes. Honest and open debate, however, is healthy because hidden agendas grow like cancers in the recesses of the enterprise.

### Setting Strategy and Prioritizing Projects

Just as some organizations bleed to death when they make a thousand cuts in hopes of making one surgically precise incision, so a leader can suffer under myriad initiatives that work at cross-purposes. Terry Neill, worldwide managing partner of Andersen Consulting's Change Management Services, calls it "death by a thousand initiatives": Employees at organizations that are changing everything from accounting systems to paper clips are likely to experience the ill effects of confusion and organizational chaos. Whereas there is value in strategically conceived disorientation, there is disaster in disarray.

Good leaders, therefore, have to make hard decisions about irrelevant or obsolete projects. They must insist on jettisoning those projects that are not aligned with the organization's objectives and critical success factors. At the beginning of an enterprise transformation, many leaders are tempted to change everything and change it radically. Effective coordination is very difficult, and as a result leaders may seek to build encouragement through incremental successes.

### Identifying "Quick Wins"

Mickey Herbert began his career in health care back in the early 1970s when he became an administrative assistant for Paul Ellwood, M.D., president of InterStudy, a health policy research firm in Minneapolis. When, during the Nixon years, the HMO Act passed (largely through lobbyists' efforts), Herbert seized the opportunity to build Physicians Health Services (PHS) from a fledgling operation with two employees into a major player in managed care. Beginning in the late 1970s with some 6,000 members, PHS expanded its enrollment by 1982 to 24,000, although even with this increase it still operated at a break-even level. With the Reagan administration cutting off funding to HMOs, Herbert began a concerted effort to acquire Fairfield Health Plan in Stamford, Connecticut, which was in danger of going out of business. This was the first of several strategic moves that drew PHS into a larger playing field, first in Connecticut, then throughout southern New England. Just two years later, in 1984, PHS became the largest HMO in Connecticut. (Herbert 1995)

Herbert determined that the success of PHS depended on expanding into the tristate region of New York, New Jersey, and Connecticut; marketing its products to a wider base; and establishing contracts with as many physicians and hospitals as possible. One consulting group predicted that PHS would need to sign up about 1,500 physicians and 30 hospitals in New York City and Long Island to be competitive. In its history of hospital and physician recruitment, PHS had developed a well-deserved reputation for effective leadership and excellent services. Herbert saw the possibility for a quick win in the New York market; accordingly, he hired a group of recruiters and put them in charge of making inroads into New York. The results were astounding: Instead of 1,500, PHS contracted with 7,500 physicians; instead of 30 hospitals, PHS got 67. (Herbert 1995).

Exemplifying the qualities of a great leader, Mickey Herbert has insisted on setting up the tangible, achievable goal, which is quantifiable and illustrates future possibilities. Unless they set specific goals, few organizations can gain all their objectives at once; most of them work incrementally, spacing out the measures of success by limiting their objectives. Sometimes, of course, these measures must change as the industry fluctuates.

In our surveys of successful health care enterprises, we also found that change can often occur more quickly in areas that are located away from corporate headquarters or regional offices. Whether it is escaping the strong gravitational pull of the central bureaucracy or feeling the freedom of exploring new areas, high-performance organizations frequently look for the opportunity to achieve immediate successes in outlying areas. For example, Mickey Herbert reports that through Paul Philpott, PHS went outside its tri-state concentration to form an alliance with The Guardian, a 130-year-old indemnity insurance company that had long-standing relationships with more than 1,000 brokers in New York. Now PHS can market its managed care product and be competitive in the rapidly changing health care environment in the largest metropolitan area in the United States. (Herbert 1995)

### Choosing Leaders and Developing Sponsors

Dick Wright of PhyCor tells a revealing story about CEO Joe Hutts when he was conceiving the new venture. Hutts had determined that he would spend six months searching for some of the giants of the industry to help him run the new company. But as time went on, he discovered that the team did not come together as he knew it should.

One evening he sat reading a book entitled *The Quest for Character* by Chuck Swindoll, who describes how Christ's twelve disciples had come together. They were a ragged aggregation of souls, but they proved to be achievers of a level that no one would have predicted. The author recommended that instead of going for the big names, it is better to look for trustworthy people, love them, cultivate their faith and friendship, and then watch God work: A team that is drawn together by love and held together by grace has staying power and the ability to grow old gracefully.

As Joe Hutts read that, he was struck by the fact that maybe his plan of action was wrong. At 10:45 p.m., Hutts called Wright to invite him to join a new team that he was conceiving. Hutts arranged a meeting for the new team next morning at 7:30, and by the following day at 5:00 p.m., they had a business plan and assigned responsibilities, and in only 23 days PhyCor had a commitment of $3 million from their initial venture capital firm. (Wright 1995)

Choosing leaders is not an exact science. As the story about Joe Hutts illustrates, it is a matter for some intuition and faith, informed by observation and personal accomplishments. When Terry White at MetroHealth needed a new vice president for human resources, he knew the job would require a person with a keen political sense, someone who could work effectively in the rapidly changing Cleveland marketplace. ("Battle for Cleveland" 1994) The ideal candidate had to know how to twist arms in some cases and how to use gentle persuasion in others. Moreover, the new vice president would have to survive in the political dogfights that were sure to occur in this environment. Surveying the field, White chose Paul Patton, who had headed up the human-resources office in Mayor Michael White's office in Cleveland. Patton's work, according to those who follow the changes in Cleveland and elsewhere, has been outstanding, and Terry White has been successful in developing sponsorship throughout MetroHealth.

The development of that sponsorship is one of the keys to the organization's success. At Allina Health System, Gordon Sprenger insisted on dropping the "C" from his title "CEO." He wanted to foster a sense of a diminishing hierarchy in the managerial ranks. Accordingly, he called on other executives to change their titles by removing those designations that create the layer cake approach to management. Currently at Allina there are no "special" assistants, "second vice presidents," or "chief officers." (Sprenger 1995) While initially drawing gasps of disbelief and scoffs of cynicism, Sprenger's proposal paid off by reducing the sense of hierarchy and creating a greater sense of equality among employees and other stakeholders in the organization. Their support for Sprenger and for each other has helped the organization withstand the growing pains that followed the 1994 merger of HMO Medica and Health Span/Health Systems Corporation, out of which Allina Health System arose. (Sprenger 1995)

Joe Hutts believes that PhyCor's success lies chiefly in its corporate culture, which encourages people to make decisions based on what they know to be right and ethical, without fear of reprisals if they make a mistake. To promote this culture, PhyCor avoids hierarchical gradations of people in the corporate organization. You won't find job titles like "senior vice president" and "assistant director" at PhyCor. The emphasis falls instead on teams of people who can work well together, no matter what rung they occupy on the corporate ladder. They sit down to work out problems and create a sense of community by bringing in anyone who can contribute to finding solutions. (Hutts 1995)

If your program for change is to succeed, you must have the support of key stakeholders throughout the organization. It's not enough just to get the approval of the executive team or the people in charge of developing products and services. It must be everyone.

This is probably the most difficult part of managing change because, as leaders everywhere can tell you, discouragement rushes in to fill the gaps left by unenthusiastic employees, partners, or customers. Leaders who fail to notice the signs of this discouragement will surely feel the pain of a failed transformation.

When Dr. Judy Lim became the CEO of Tan Tock Seng Hospital in Singapore in 1991, she found the worst case of low morale and poor self-esteem among staff members that she had ever seen. Dispirited and disappointed, hospital employees expressed deep fears of change even though they thought their present conditions intolerable. Lim saw in the dilapidated physical plant an apt image of everyone's state of mind, and she resolved to revive their desire for excellence and to awaken the dormant sense of self-respect. She knew this would be no easy task: She had to persuade the staff that it was worse to remain where they were than to attempt to move to higher ground.

Largely through her personal commitment to the hospital staff and the change program, Lim reversed this downward trend. Initially, she had to embody the vision by herself as she worked to fire up her people with the new ideas. She recognized that success ultimately required ensuring that every single staff member understood and was equally committed to the same mission and vision. To accomplish this, they needed to understand the journey destination and receive satisfaction and personal fulfillment during the change process. To quickly generate enthusiasm, she installed new information technology that would really empower employees and implemented flattened authority and decision-making processes and structures. She started in the intensive care units, and the innovation had immediate effects in the delivery of excellent care. Furthermore, the system attracted the attention of health care organizations throughout Southeast Asia. In addition, the hospital began converting burdensome paper files into electronic patient records, first for its intensive care patients, then for outpatients. In a little more than six months, Tan Tock Seng Hospital introduced technological innovations that helped to jump-start employees' attitudes. Lim sees her role at Tan Tock Seng as akin to that of a missionary: "You have to preach all the time, but even more important, you have to practice what you preach so that people can see that it is not just a pipe dream but a goal that we can actually achieve." (Lim 1995)

David Campbell at St. Vincent's would agree. "You do not change any organization," he says, "unless you have incredible courage, persistence, and key supporters who are willing to share the vision and not take you down when things get tough. You have to make sure that you have adequate support when you bring about major change, from the owners, the shareholders, and the board." (Campbell 1995)

Sponsors need to be cultivated and trained. It is not enough just to give them the charge and communicate with them once in a while to inquire how things are going. The most successful change programs are those in which people throughout the organization invest heavily, not just their time and loyalty, but also their creative energy and thinking. It's a bank account from which one does not withdraw funds;

rather, the invested resources bring in more investments from more and more employees.

When they begin to develop a sense of ownership, employees themselves take the initiative for seeing projects go forward. Recognizing the potential of that sense, managers at Vanderbilt University Medical Center in Nashville, Tennessee, recently began offering a three-day course in "facilitative leadership." (Sherer 1994: 42) The facilitative leader par excellence, Gordon Sprenger simply laid the cards out on the table when he told laboratory personnel that Allina had to reduce lab costs by several million dollars. He could have proclaimed how these reductions would be achieved, but instead he presented the results he wanted. The laboratory personnel went to work and came up with their own strategy for achieving the reduction.

Surely, this must be what Dwight D. Eisenhower meant when he observed that "leadership is the art of getting someone else to do something you want done because he [or she] wants to do it."

### Executing the Plan

Many a great plan of action has been formulated and launched, only to be lost in the execution. Whether caused by a failure of nerve, a lack of conviction, or a fault of will, the inability to follow through with tenacity and sympathy has spelled doom for many corporate executives and their organizations.

### Demonstrating Personal Commitment

Unless leaders and their executive teams are willing to change their behaviors and daily activities to bring them in line with the vision, others in the corporation will quickly lose the enthusiasm for change. Nowhere is the old adage of practicing what you preach more applicable than in managing the complex transformation of a large enterprise. Terry White, for example, put his own reputation at risk when he voluntarily left a successful job in Cincinnati to take a more challenging job in Cleveland. Now at MetroHealth, White has created a corporate culture oriented to a strong sense of ethics, a set of core values to which everyone in the organization must adhere, no matter what job they perform. He believes that senior management and physicians must always be aware of what the other side is doing and that no one should cut special deals with the CEO. When he is blindsided, he admits the mistake in judgment and moves quickly to correct it.

As an example of his personal commitment to change, White acknowledges that having established a committee to allocate capital equipment and space, he himself once attempted to do an end run around those managers: "I got myself into a corner because I decided on my own that I was going to move data processing to another part of the facility, but I failed to clear this with the very committee I had set up to monitor the use of physical space. Somebody asked me if I was serious about this committee. That's when I realized that I had erred and done the very thing that disturbed me about the way the organization used to be run." (White 1995)

### Aligning Rewards and Taking Reality Checks

Every change program requires some change in behavior: People simply cannot work the way they used to. Whether beginning a new diet or redesigning an organization's internal processes, change is hard. Every behavior modification requires some reward for sacrifice.

In aligning rewards, however, we often find a paradox in human behavior: Whereas those doing the work respond better to positive reinforcement, it is often the case that those assessing the work find it easier to criticize than to praise. Like the math teacher who always marked the incorrect responses on the test, many corporate leaders focus on what went wrong rather than on what was done correctly and productively. They seem unable to praise employees when they complete a task in ways that the leaders had not anticipated.

Gordon Sprenger is a leader who has an intuitive sense for drawing the best out of people. Rather than designating himself as the corporate czar, he prefers the designations "coach" and "main strategist" for the organization. Surrounding himself with the best people, he inspires them by promoting trust and freedom, rewarding them for working well in collaborative relationships, and removing the traditional hierarchical designations that work against the productivity that peers can achieve. Like Gail Warden at Henry Ford Health System, Sprenger believes in bringing together representative customers to help create the company's strategy by asking where Allina needs to go and what it needs to do to get there. With a deeper sense of ownership in the change process, those sponsors take on the responsibility of ensuring that the transformation continues in productive ways.

### Sustaining the Change

The quickest way to kill a transformation program is to leave it alone once it has been put in place. Entropy, the tendency for systems to wind down and lose momentum, applies equally to forces that occur in nature and to operations that human beings create. Even burning platforms will flame out if they are left to their own devices; of course, the destruction they leave is deadly.

Great leaders intuitively recognize that danger or they have seen its effects in other transformation projects they have directed.

## Assessing and Refining the Change

Without periodic reality checks, you cannot accurately assess the change program you have put in place, nor can you make those alterations—minute or massive—that keep the organization robust. Gail Warden sends his CEO's letter to all employees at the end of each year, reminding them that pressures in the health care industry continue to increase and that reducing costs is paramount to the future success of Henry Ford Health System. Although it is not a popular note to sound, he speaks frankly in this "Year-End Usage" letter about the need to keep a lid on salaries. (Warden 1995) Taking another tack, Terry White meets with the management team at MetroHealth every Tuesday and opens his door for an hour or more each week to any manager who wants to discuss an issue that is related to the organization.

Whatever schedule you choose, you need to announce it publicly and follow it consistently. Wherever appropriate, leaders of the transformation program offer objective measures of progress and outcomes, comparing them with the objectives that they established in the planning and launching process. If you and your management team detect a lack of progress in one or more areas, you can investigate its causes and try to correct it before it undermines the entire transformation program. If you would refuse to allow a tumor to remain in place and possibly metastasize, why would you turn your gaze away from the cancers in your organization's body?

## Removing Barriers

Good leaders have zero tolerance for barriers that stand in the way of progress in the transformation. If your heart skips a beat for the loss of that 1958 Cadillac, then you are probably going to have problems sustaining the change initiative you've put in place. The effective leader surveys the entire organization with an eye toward removing any block, regardless of whether it is a particular individual who resists change completely, a company policy that has solidified itself into iron law, or a department that has built such high walls around its functions that it determines how the rest of the organization conducts business.

Some leaders approach the task with a ruthless blade; others take a more delicate approach, fully aware that astute politicking can reduce resistance better than slash-and-burn tactics. When he took over as CEO, David Campbell recognized that for nearly a century St. Vincent's Hospital had been inspired by the strongly held values of the Sisters of Charity. Changing to a more secular culture and injecting business practices that took a more realistic view of the rapidly changing Australian health care industry required a delicate touch rather than iron-fisted declamation.

Gail Warden, on the other hand, came to Henry Ford Health Care Corporation in 1988 and counted 22 different cultures, pension plans, and salary schedules, which he describes as hanging like lights on a Christmas tree. By introducing total quality management (TQM), Warden began a major reorientation project that would bring everyone together under the single light of the Henry Ford Health System. Uniting independent physicians and corporate administrators (two groups that in the past have rarely seen health care issues in the same way), Warden built a new culture that stresses the continuum of care from birth to death. He directed the leadership team to scrutinize the 1,200 vacancies that the change program had created in the organization and to determine which ones could be eliminated. After effectively consolidating processes and clearly communicating the need for these changes, the leadership team eliminated 700 positions without reducing staff. (Warden 1995)

Sustaining a change program requires a leader who can act decisively to remove any barrier that stands in the way of the organization's progress. If this barrier happens to be an employee, a great leader's respectful treatment of the individual will demonstrate sympathy (not sentimentality) and help the employee retain self-esteem and a sense of value. Mickey Herbert at PHS illustrates this standard of ethics. He believes that if there are decent, talented people in the organization— people who are willing to work hard and who show initiative— there are places they can fit in. He recounts the case of an introverted employee who much preferred working in front of a desktop computer to dealing directly with physicians. Easily intimidated by high-powered doctors, this man was ill-suited to direct one of PHS's entrepreneurial sites, but Herbert found a perfect position for him in the claims department where he has become a critical player in the company's operations. (Herbert 1995)

Managing the complex transformation of today's health care enterprise will quickly identify for you the strengths and weaknesses you and your organization have. Planning and launching such a change requires imaginative minds that can organize and delegate responsibility, rapidly survey a system in disarray, and invent a new structure that will set the enterprise on the way to success. Enacting those changes is more difficult: That part of the transforming process takes deeply personal commitment and the ability to infuse that sense of excitement into everyone else in the organization. Not surprisingly, these are often people who have known only one way of doing their jobs and who are fearful of change. Sustaining the transformation is probably the toughest of all. Not only does it require the talents and qualities mentioned above, but also it takes courage and tenacity.

# REFERENCES

"The Battle for Cleveland." *Integrated Healthcare Report.* September, 1994: 1–8.

Campbell, David. 1995. Interview with Kurt Miller. Melbourne, Australia.

Conner, Darryl. 1992. *Managing at the speed of change: how resilient managers succeed and prosper where others fail.* New York: Villard Books.

Flower, Joe. 1995. Leadership without easy answers. *Healthcare Forum,* July–August: 30–36.

Herbert, Mickey. 1995. Interview with Ken Jennings, Wendy Kingsbury, and Ian Galliot. Hartford, Connecticut. October 17.

Hutts, Joe. 1995. Interview with David Osborne and Mike Raney.

Lim, Judy. 1995. Interview with Kurt Miller. Singapore.

Peters, Tom. 1987. *Thriving on chaos: handbook for a management revolution.* New York: HarperCollins.

Reinertsen, James L. 1994. Beyond process improvement. Presentation to the Sixth Annual National Forum on Quality Improvement in Health Care. San Diego, Calif.

Sherer, Jill L. 1993. Structure follows strategy. *Hospitals & Health Networks,* November 5: 22–28.

———1994. Retooling leaders: "facilitative leadership" helps clarify process and underpin culture change. *Hospitals & Health Networks,* January 5: 42, 44.

Sprenger, Gordon. 1995. Interview with Ken Jennings.

Understanding the enterprise transformation journey. 1995. Unpublished report. Andersen Consulting. May 12.

Warden, Gail. 1995. Interview with Ken Jennings. Detroit, Michigan.

White, Terry R. 1995. Interview with Ken Jennings. Cleveland, Ohio.

Wright, Dick. 1995. Interview with Ken Jennings and Erik Hansen.

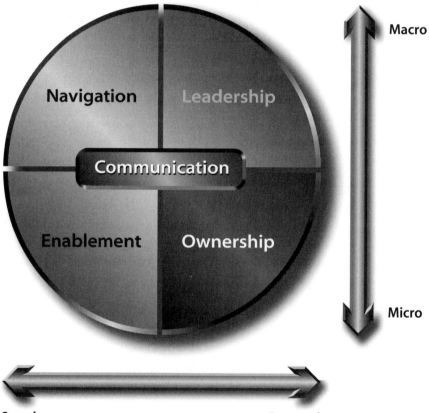

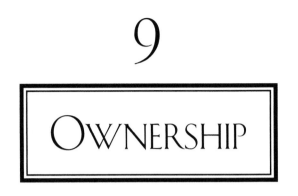

# 9

# OWNERSHIP

Robert Fusco, president of Olsten Kimberly Quality-Care, has fashioned an astonishing vision for his corporation. He foresees the radical transformation of his $1.3-billion firm, the largest provider of home health care in North America, into an integrated health care organization. In his brave new picture of the future, the niche company that now offers a narrow menu of home health services—skilled nursing, physical therapy, rehabilitative care, infusion therapy, hospice care, paramedic services—will be gone. The new Olsten will offer the best of the past, namely, outstanding nursing, along with a broader menu of health care services.

Fusco puts his objective simply: "We will own the process of managing care." (Fusco 1996: 4) He aims to redefine his company's present identification: "In five years," he says, "I don't want to be looked at as a home health care service company." (Fusco 1996: 4)

He plans to realize this vision in two steps. First, he will turn the company into a home health care manager, responsible not only for nursing but also for costs, quality, utilization, administration, and financial risk. Second, he will turn the company into a manager that integrates and coordinates all care seamlessly.

To get Olsten Kimberly QualityCare to that point, Fusco knows he must convince his people to share his vision as a creation they themselves help to build. They must rally around the strategies and objectives for realizing that vision, and they must zealously apply their own skills to deliver the sustained performance that will make the vision a reality.

Fusco has taken a leadership role in getting his people to own this vision. Like other executives managing change programs, he knows that the job of building ownership is the keystone to success. Those stakeholders who resist change can sabotage the entire venture by ignoring critical strategies and objectives. They will try to prove their bosses wrong at every turn. Although they may put in time at their desks, the resisters will bog down change in thousands of intractable ways.

That is why a methodical approach to developing ownership is so important. From our interviews and experience working with health enterprises, we have found that gaining ownership requires a program with three prime elements:

▼ *A change network:* A shadow organization of employee champions, advocates, and coaches to spur transformation.

▼ *A communication plan:* A strategy and schedule for both delivering change messages and getting feedback on an organization-wide level.

▼ *A method for local action:* Tools, techniques, and skills for solving problems and affecting change in every local unit.

Fusco's work at Olsten Kimberly QualityCare offers a snapshot of all three. The prime agents of change at Olsten are the members of the so-called Network Development Team, executives charged with moving Olsten through the first stage of its transformation, from a vendor of home health care services to a manager of home health care networks. This executive team has, in turn, named six coteams—in the areas of finance, operations, provider relations, business development, strategic development, and information systems—that will establish the processes, systems, and infrastructure of the expanded business. (Olsten Kimberly 1996a)

To communicate the change program, Fusco constructed a road map that employed colorful graphics to present the principles that will guide Olsten on its journey to an integrated health care organization. As employees and other stakeholders unfold the map, they find it details the company's mission, vision, shared values, balanced scorecard measures, and behaviors consistent with the company's values. (Olsten Kimberly 1996b)

To spur local action, Olsten strengthened the skills and procedures associated with quality management and organized Olsten to operate with a team structure. Indeed, Fusco even established a team to reengineer all of the policies, procedures, and processes in the company's 600 branch offices. The results of this reengineering, called the Gold Standard, created more uniform, efficient, and customer-friendly processes. Now every branch runs itself the same way when it comes to everything from scheduling and records management to payroll and quality improvement. (Olsten Kimberly 1996a)

Olsten is a good example of how ownership programs can yield a speedy payback. Less than a year after the executive team began its work, both Aetna and Cigna Healthcare signed huge contracts with the company. Olsten Kimberly Quality-Care now manages all of the home health care needs for these two managed care giants. Cigna alone brought to Olsten nearly ten million HMO and PPO members and a contract valued at up to $100 million in revenues over three years. (Olsten 1996; Olsten Kimberly 1996a) With the large Cigna and Aetna contracts, Fusco transported his company out of the role of a mere vendor. He coaxed customers themselves, voting with huge contract dollars, to consider Olsten a network manager, a partner with the payer.

"Defined today, you can look at our network management business as a single benefit HMO," says Fusco. "We are managing the entire spectrum of home health care for large payers." (Fusco 1996)

A successful transformation at that scale demands that top managers strive to develop a feeling of ownership that runs both wide and deep. Organizations in the process of change need buy-in from people at every level. The ownership program must bring on board every group, every manager, every professional. Ownership, however, must go well beyond perfunctory buy-in. The ownership program must turn every underground group of resistance and indifference into fervent supporters.

The goal of ownership programs, in other words, is to gain commitment that spontaneously stirs people to grasp the vision and organizational objectives, to take responsibility for change, to exercise all of their professional energies, and to contribute their most valuable insights to guiding the organization on the road to the future. When top managers succeed in developing true ownership, they find that the organization solves problems far more rapidly and meets priority business objectives far sooner. It thus leaves imitators and competitors in the dust.

## Building the Change Network

In building ownership, executives need to direct, coordinate, and support the change network. Whereas today's organization structures itself in a hierarchy of managers who oversee products and services (with an occasional foray into process management), the creation of the new organization must be directed by a separate structure comprising sponsors, change agents, and change advocates. Some of the managers holding the reins of power in today's organization will also hold them in the change network, but more often a separate group of people will be dedicated to the task.

The change network begins small—a team of five to fifty change agents—then expands to embrace more people at each level of the organization. By selling the change at all levels, the change network quickly gains a critical mass of support, winning the acceptance of and personal responsibility for the change by people throughout the organization.

The function of the change network resembles that of a marketing and distribution organization for a new product: It retrieves information from the consumers of change, namely, the employees, and then markets, promotes, and distributes the programs of change based on the expectations of these customers.

Although akin to a marketing and distribution system, the change network is not a command-and-control hierarchy that simply fills old communications pipelines with stale change messages. In fact, traditional hierarchical communication channels work poorly to promote the flow of information and knowledge necessary for successful change. Within the change network, knowledge and information must flow simultaneously from the top down, from the bottom up, and from side to side. Top-down information helps coordinate organizational efforts from headquarters management. Bottom-up information assists top management in measuring the progress of change, identifying glitches, and taking the pulse of employee attitudes and expectations. Lateral communication—the most deficient in hierarchical organizations—promotes the sharing of best practices.

The network's most important task extends well beyond mere communication. It extends to involving people at every level in the change. Employees must participate in everything from the formulation of strategy to the fine-tuning of programs aimed at changing their work groups—their attitudes, their behaviors, and their vision for the future. A high level of involvement creates a culture of individual accountability and problem solving. In the best cases, it turns every employee into a change advocate.

To initiate change, top managers must first craft a design that fits the organization, articulates the network's mission, and defines the speed of change, the means of achieving it, and the measures of success. Next, they must identify the divisions, groups, and people targeted for change; what their competencies, values, and behaviors are; and where they are located throughout the company. Because the network establishes new hierarchy and new communication channels alongside the existing channels, top managers must delineate how the two relate and how the two can be integrated once the change project winds down.

Developing the change network requires identifying each organizational niche that needs an agent of change. Managers pinpoint change agents at the local level first, then add supervisors to oversee the knowledge exchange. In most cases, the supervisory span of control should not exceed fifteen people. Ideally, the change network should operate with no more than three levels to expedite the flow of information throughout the network. A change network manager can control the center, while central change agents, intermediate change agents, and local change agents sell the change directly into the local units.

The role of change agents varies with the circumstances and with their level in the organization. Most frequently, change agents in local units act as facilitators, generating enthusiasm for the change and utilizing their skills and expertise to help make the change happen. Meanwhile, the supervisors of change agents apply pressure to make the change happen expeditiously. Acting together, people in the change network will use both carrots and sticks to get people's attention and help them migrate into the roles that will support the organization's future vision.

Choosing the right people is, of course, essential to the success of the change network. The best change agents are those who communicate well, who work well with others, who know their way around the organization, its culture, rules, and processes. They are committed to change and enjoy strong credibility among superiors, peers, and subordinates— enough to speak for inventing a new future and burying (with all due respect) the past.

After several years of incremental improvements, Kaiser Permanente Southern California Region took a systematic approach to creating a change network when it set out to reengineer its core administrative processes in 1995. Working with Jon Rands, Zach Brooks, and Paige Heavey of Andersen Consulting, Kaiser Permanente first identified the hundreds of stakeholder groups, from patient accounting and regional collections to pharmacy operations and admitting, to family practice physicians and hospital administrators. The HMO then created the change network, naming executives, midlevel sponsors, and local agents, including receptionists, clerks, nurses, and physicians.

Kaiser Permanente sought to involve people throughout the organization at every stage of the reengineering, from design and training to implementation. Managers identified many change agents during the design phase and asked them what kind of training they needed as well as what rewards they expected. The change team filmed receptionists to create training videos and published their testimonials about the change; it even held a pizza party to celebrate results. The involvement created buy-in and ownership where the organization might otherwise have stumbled on resistance.

A particularly important opportunity for building ownership comes when the change network contracts with business units to finance the new programs. Who will pay the bulk of the costs? Who will be involved? How will success be measured? Negotiations to pin down these details, identify the change agents, and debate the measures of success all offer opportunities to build ownership.

The monitoring system and the evolving network deserve special consideration. In addition to gauging performance according to specified goals, the monitoring system details how the network reports results, tracks progress not captured by a fixed set of indicators, and feeds information back to the network to foster knowledge-sharing, organizational learning, and continuous improvement. Some organizations use scorecards of progress, network meetings, electronic question-and-answer bulletin boards, and a change network war room for planning quick changes and rallying team spirit.

The plan for expanding the change network must be put in place even before it is launched. Although the network begins with a team of a half dozen top executives, it will expand downward through the organizational hierarchy, recruiting new change agents at every step and detailing how it will expand into various functions and geographies. Anticipating eventual completion, change mangers also outline the merging of the network with the ongoing hierarchy of the organization or the disbanding of the network when it has outlived its usefulness.

Generally, the network helps the organization change in phases, moving gradually to define people's roles, allocate funds, provide training, and specify the techniques for achieving buy-in. Change managers also celebrate interim accomplishments in highly visible ways.

### The Communication Plan

The second critical element in building ownership is a plan for communicating. Ultimately the plan seeks to move the organization from the awareness of a need for change to acceptance, support, and commitment. The plan serves as a continuously changing guidebook of strategies, tactics, and methods necessary for organization-wide communication. Accordingly, it details four steps: preparation, development, execution, and evaluation.

A distinguishing feature of effective communication planning is that it engages people in change rather than simply telling them about it. Accordingly, the communication must flow in two directions. Managers detail the changes for people throughout the organization, who then have an opportunity to respond and evaluate the changes before, during, and after they occur. Communication must become an active and open dialogue. When Kaiser Permanente Southern California Region developed its communication plan, it both created this dialogue and involved people in every step of the planning. It developed focus groups of employees at all levels and encouraged them to speak frankly about the effectiveness of the change initiatives.

The change management team must clearly articulate the plan's objectives, build trust, minimize resistance, and create a sense of enthusiastic ownership. For example, executives at St. Ann's Hospital in Columbus, Ohio, embarked on a radical transformation in 1993. Their goal was to slash costs by a remarkable 50 percent while improving the quality of care. Their plan was to restructure seventy-two departments and cost centers into fourteen care and support centers, encourage communication vertically and horizontally in the hospital, help staff manage the change, and maintain consistency with corporate culture.

A third element of the successful communication plan is identifying, assessing, and segmenting key audiences within the organization. If the product being sold is change itself, the sponsors and agents of change must determine how best to reach the customers they want to buy the product. When Kaiser Permanente Southern California Region set out to create a communication plan, it questioned hundreds of people and inventoried functions and positions throughout the organization that would be affected by change. It then segmented these stakeholders into groups according to unique communication needs. Before developing any communication programs, the HMO's change team evaluated each stakeholder group to obtain and understand its history of change, level of commitment, and perspectives on Kaiser Permanente.

One stakeholder group, for example, included the frontline employees—receptionists, cashiers, and admitting clerks. The assessment showed that many of them thought the intention of the change was to cut their salaries or eliminate their jobs. When they heard that Kaiser was proposing to create new positions, many deduced that the added expenses for these jobs would come out of their salaries. "There goes my raise," commented one of the participants in a kickoff meeting. Although such comments stemmed only from rumors, they revealed to Kaiser managers the work they had to do in developing an effective communication plan, one that would quell concerns of the frontline staff.

No matter how simple or complex the message, the organization needs to look closely at its channels for communicating with stakeholders. Some organizations rely chiefly on newsletters; others, on e-mail and memos. At Kaiser Permanente, the assessment revealed that a number of channels—newsletters, staff meetings, e-mail, internal magazines, and employee forums—would be useful for distributing messages to employees and gathering feedback. It also revealed the deficiencies in the communications system that needed to be corrected.

And however sophisticated the channels of communication, they are worthless if the organization does not encourage discussion and debate about the transformation. From the start, managers must involve all employees in the change. How they do it—through focus groups, town meetings, face-to-face interviews, or internal surveys—is less important than the perception that stakeholders' views are taken seriously and that the discussion is not just a perfunctory exercise after the executive team has already decided what changes must occur.

At MetroHealth in Cleveland, Ohio, CEO Terry White invited all employees to contribute to the organization's strategic plan. Although an executive team shaped the plan, White sent copies to all employees to request ongoing feedback for subsequent planning. "The function of strategic planning is not simply to produce a document," he told employees. "It is a process by which we build consensus about what we wish to do and how we wish to do it." ("Vision 2000" 1994)

Similarly, Allina Health System CEO Gordon Sprenger consistently adheres to a philosophy of bringing the entire organization into the process of setting strategy. "You create strategy, you don't design it," he says. "By creating it, I mean you engage the organization in the creation of it. . . . We, together, create that strategy." (Sprenger 1995)

When Allina began looking at ways to improve community health, for example, each member of Sprenger's top management group participated in as many as eight focus groups with people from throughout the organization, roughly 600 in all. The executives tested their ideas with the employees, drawing out concerns, assessing opportunities, and predicting customers' reactions. All of the employees, as well as the company's labor-management council and physician committees, helped shape the final vision. (Howe 1995) "We underestimate the imaginativeness and the creativity of our workforce; it's immense," says Sprenger. "They will create not only strategies, but also tactics. Through their participation, employees develop a greater sense of ownership." (Sprenger 1995)

In developing the change plan itself, executives must articulate key messages, highlighting those that are important to certain segments of the audience. Second, they must identify the most appropriate channels for delivering information and retrieving feedback. Third, they need to prioritize and schedule events, programs, and activities.

For example, executives at St. Ann's Hospital in Columbus, Ohio, began the development of the change plan by publicizing the need to maintain or improve quality while reducing costs: "St. Ann's must change to secure its future"; "Change will benefit patients, staff, and physicians"; and "St. Ann's will be prepared for health care industry changes." The change network then created a series of matrices to detail communication for each of its audiences: staff, physicians, board members, employees, volunteers, patients, payers, donors, and the media. Each matrix listed communication vehicles, objectives, frequency, dates, locations, and feedback mechanisms.

The key objectives included building trust, awareness, and two-way communication. To accomplish these, the change management team held monthly question and answer sessions in the hospital cafeteria, which proved to be a successful means of building staff morale and ownership. The team also established a toll-free telephone number for collecting employee questions, frequent departmental presentations, a communication team consisting of representatives from every shift and department, and various social and sports events to increase the interaction of the team with the employees.

Once the employees take hold of the plan, it is much easier to follow through with the execution. The execution of many large communication plans starts with a kickoff event. At St. Ann's, the CEO and CFO adopted the town meeting format, a hospital tradition, to convey the especially sensitive information about the change directly to everyone involved. In the increasingly competitive world of health care, the CEO at the time, Jack Sandman, told employees that everyone's job was at risk, even his own. His statement proved prophetic when he left the hospital after its acquisition by Mount Carmel Health Care in 1995. Because change brings such serious consequences, managers must offer face-to-face communication. Employees need to hear the argument for change, the consequences of not changing, and the benefits that the change will bring. And they need to hear it over and over. MetroHealth's Terry White likes to recount a backhanded compliment he once received regarding the way he communicates: "One of my former associates, who went on to become a CEO, said I am the most boring person he ever worked with because I say the same thing over and over. I say it to the board, to the leadership team, to the medical staff, to the employees. He got so sick of hearing me say the same thing ten different ways to people." (White 1995)

The St. Ann's team came up with an innovative means of eliciting response. Called the Grape Vine (some employees dubbed it the Gripe Vine), this bulletin board gives employees a place to post rumors they have heard about the changes at the hospital. Managers respond to these postings by rebutting, explaining, or confirming them. For the first year and a half of change, the Vine flourished with postings. Not only did it squelch rumors, but it also gave employees a chance to vent their feelings and to debate change issues with disenchanted employees. Their participation helped them achieve a greater sense of ownership. (Brennan 1995)

Communication planning also requires realistic and accurate evaluation. Some of this assessment comes from informal feedback, but most of it must rely on a system to measure performance and improve communications by identifying and correcting weaknesses in the change program. The goal is to review progress against budget and scheduling targets as well as measure progress in effective communication of change messages. Evaluating feedback should be an open process, like the rest of communication planning. The organization publicizes the responses and the changes that result from them. It asks employees to help solve communication problems, to suggest modifications to communication strategy, and to brainstorm new means of communication that engender ownership. Communication planning, therefore, becomes another element in the process of organizational learning: learning how to perform at a high level in a new world.

### Creating Local Action

The third critical element in building ownership should be the creation of a method for making change happen in every group in the organization. Despite the presence of the change network and a communication plan, people at or near the front lines will rarely embrace change without specific means to change their attitudes, goals, behaviors, and the way they work. The goal is not to find a way to steamroll people into compliance; rather, it seeks to introduce the methods, tools, and techniques to help people make the change themselves.

The first step, then, in creating local action is to redefine success for every employee affected by change. That means translating the overarching targets and measures for the organization into targets and measures meaningful at the local level. Some organizations call this process cascading measurement. The largest organizational units set targets first, then the next largest sets targets, and so on down to the individuals themselves. At each level, people setting the targets must take responsibility for achieving them, but at the same time it is essential that these are "stretch" targets.

As the word *stretch* implies, these targets should press the organization into stretching its performance beyond its traditional ambitions. St. Ann's Hospital offered a clear example when executives announced that expenses had to be cut by 50 percent. Although they knew this target might not be achievable, they recognized that the organization had to do better than the 8 to 12 percent saved in other services organizations.

Faced with the challenge to reduce expenses by 50 percent, the team at St. Ann's had to look at every possibility for savings, including deleting or modifying favorite projects such as those that provided funding for scholarships, athletic programs, and nursing programs at a local college. The project team initially identified a new operational design that would reduce their total annual expenses by 24 to 48 percent at a cost of $36 to $100 million. Though still shy of the goal, they inventoried further sources of savings. In the end, the executive team revised its initial stretch target, choosing from its inventory of cuts a still hefty goal of cutting 24 percent of costs. This 24 percent target was the most they could afford to finance and was expected to position them as the lowest-cost, highest-quality hospital in the area.

Targets should be quantifiable. Not all, of course, lend themselves to numeric measures, but whenever possible, the organization should set them so that the achievements suffer as little distortion as possible from subjective assessments. To keep the measurement system practical, the measures of targets should, wherever possible, depend on data the organization already produces. The standard 80/20 rule usually applies: At least 80 percent of the data needed to measure success should be easy to come by; the other 20 percent will require new ways to capture and report performance.

As in all other aspects of developing ownership, coming up with targets and measures of success must result from thorough debate and deliberation within the organization. Employees subjected to measures must have their say in how they are developed. The discussion will build employees' confidence that the organization is listening to them and that their ideas are valued. It also helps people gain a better understanding of how the measures at their level connect to measures at the next and how they in turn all contribute to the organization's future. Should managers dictate measures, rather than allow widespread deliberation, they will find that people simply do not buy into the new definition of success.

Inspiring local action, the targets should offer a measure of business outcomes, progress in implementing ownership programs, and acceptance of the degree of ownership that results. At the organizational level, for example, St. Ann's developed business measures that gauge financial performance, care quality, and satisfaction for employees, customers, and physicians. (Brennan 1995) Groups within St. Ann's translated these measures so that, at the level of care centers, budget variance and care path variance became measures. In the evaluation of care teams, the number of infections and missed procedures was used as two of several measures of performance. These measures cascaded downward, ultimately being tied to measures for frontline employees and the design of an incentive compensation system.

Organizations will have to take a similar cascading approach to developing measures for the progress of implementing ownership programs. At the top level, managers can track spending, the launching of initiatives, and the timely achievement of milestones. At the lowest levels, groups can track recruitment of change agents, training in new skills, and redesign of individual jobs.

Measuring the actual progress in building ownership will be more difficult because it calls for innovative methods of evaluation, many of which cannot be quantified. To spur local action, however, the organization should institute a variety of ways to gauge whether people are buying into the change.

Along with redefining success, organizations must facilitate action at the local level by giving people some structure in performing tasks that help make the change happen. In the past the favorite method was TQM, or total quality management, which provides various procedures for solving problems and continuously improving products and services throughout the transformation. Without some guidance, employees cannot make the necessary changes in their behaviors, jobs, and work processes. As Allina CEO Gordon Sprenger says, "The whole quality improvement process gets people mentoring each other and looking for ways to improve. You really build that into the culture of the organization. It just becomes part of the fabric of the organization. This is the way we do business." (Sprenger 1995) Whatever method an organization develops for spurring local action, it must involve employees in the work, provide them with an opportunity to experiment, value innovative ideas, give people the authority to act and the responsibility for accounting for their performance, and offer them a protected environment for mistakes.

To speed change and develop ownership, high-performing organizations are redesigning the way their teams work. Not only have team members adopted practices such as quality management, they have cross-trained to develop more skills and to take on new roles that broaden their perspectives. They work more flexibly with teammates, focusing on solving problems rather than doing jobs or defending their turf. And they strive to communicate more clearly with other teams as well as other parts of their organizations.

High-performing teams need collaborative skills to solve problems, and change managers will have to budget the funds and time to give employees this training. Gordon Sprenger reports, "We at Allina Health Services learned that we need to take time up front to train people how to be good team members. We also learned we need to send in a facilitator to help teams establish the ground rules as to how they would operate." (Sprenger 1995)

Allina now operates with self-managing teams at multiple levels. Building on an earlier example, Sprenger notes that management charged a team comprising the heads of all of Allina's clinical laboratories with cutting several million dollars of lab costs. Although Sprenger and other executives believed that the solution was to consolidate, they didn't offer that or any other alternative up front as the answer. Instead, they told the team only the amount of savings required. "The team members came back and said, 'The only way we can do this is if we centralize,'" Sprenger recalls. The lab chiefs sketched out a plan to centralize core laboratories and decentralize staff laboratories, all built around a maximum four-hour turnaround time. "Now it's their idea!" Sprenger reports happily.

Organizations that are successful with local action support their efforts by redesigning individual jobs, creating incentive systems tied to achieving targets, and establishing programs for recognition and celebration of successes. Still the most important is building skills in coaching. Practiced adeptly, coaching accelerates change.

Coaching must begin at the highest level. As Sprenger says, "I see myself as the coach and the enabler to allow people to carry out the strategy and the vision. You don't have to have a tiering of senior versus junior. Everybody knows who's got the greatest skills and the greatest competencies." (Sprenger 1995) As we noted in Chapter 8, Sprenger deleted the word "chief" from his title in an attempt to send this message to other executives and to employees: Collaboration goes further toward making an organization competitive than a dictatorship does. Executives and employees must coach each other if the organization is to succeed.

Whether executives or frontline team leaders, coaches play at least five different roles. They emphasize lessons learned, point out weak points or blind spots, reinforce successes, help develop leadership and communication skills in others, and help transfer innovations from one part of the organization to another. Coaches accelerate learning and help weave a web of rapid innovation capabilities across the organization.

We believe that effective coaches offer leadership, communication, training, consulting, problem-solving, and feedback skills. The skills of a coach are basic but vital for building the ownership model that we outline here:

▼ *Active listening:* Coaches listen both to what people say and to what they do not say. They strain to discern hints that suggest low confidence or poor commitment. To ensure proper understanding, they rephrase and repeat people's comments to gain agreement on what was said.

▼ *Questioning:* Coaches ask open-ended questions to allow people freedom to answer in their own way. Thus, they obtain information, establish rapport, and clarify and stimulate thinking. Coaches avoid leading questions or questions that insinuate fault or criticism.

▼ *Praising:* Coaches offer compliments to build self-esteem and high performance. The praise must be genuine. If it is delivered publicly, so much the better. (Conversely, fault-finding is best done in private.)

▼ *Building rapport:* Coaches overcome resistance and distrust by concentrating on common ground. They make an effort to adjust even their speech patterns to match those of the people around them.

▼ *Building trust:* Coaches build trust through reliability, openness, and sensitivity. They try to enhance other people's needs for a sense of connectedness and integrity. Coaches increase their reputation for trustworthiness by disclosing in a sensitive way their perceptions of another's behavior.

▼ *Being nonjudgmental:* Coaches disassociate themselves from their own emotions and feelings. By staying uninvolved emotionally, they allow others to form their own conclusions independently. They balance personal and management judgment, remaining open to behaviors and decisions that run against the grain of their own experience.

▼ *Being candid and challenging:* Coaches speak out frankly to draw attention to issues of benefit to others. They neither threaten nor confront; instead they phrase questions that prompt other people to challenge themselves.

▼ *Working from other people's agendas:* Coaches start by figuring out what other people want and care about. They temporarily set aside their own goals to understand those of the people they're dealing with.

▼ *Giving encouragement and support:* Coaches encourage and support others in thinking through their commitment to action. They make sure, however, that the actions of others reflect professed commitment.

▼ *Focusing on future opportunities:* Coaches focus attention on what other people would like to see happen in the future. They avoid unproductive postmortems of past efforts; instead, they encourage people to think positively about future scenarios.

▼ *Getting to the point:* Coaches intervene to clarify issues or bring discussions to a vote. They take action when a person is avoiding an issue.

▼ *Observing:* Coaches observe the whole person. They note voice, phraseology, body language, and facial expression.

Early in the program of building ownership, every organization should prepare an analysis of coaches' roles and their training needs. Without finely honed coaching skills, local action will go slowly. Although the organization may have installed mechanisms for creating ownership, the human element will be missing. It is, after all, humans who must change. Coaches who are skilled in human relations can make the transformation go much more smoothly.

Putting together all the necessary pieces to create ownership—from the change network to the communication plan, to a team-based method for local action—can seem overwhelming to employees. But the effort is essential. Olsten Kimberly QualityCare's Bob Fusco illustrates this point when he asks a question on the lips of many CEOs: "Are we doing too much, too quickly, too soon? Can I get the organization through all of this change?" (Fusco 1996) Some chief executives would say the answer is mandating change from the top. Not Fusco. "It is," he says simply, "making believers out of people."

# REFERENCES

Brennan, Jim. 1995. Interview with Susan Vanderpool. Columbus, Ohio.

Fusco, Robert. 1996. Interview with Ken Jennings, Sharyn Materna, and Mike Rainey.

Howe, Mike. 1995. Interview with Susan Vanderpool. Minnealpolis, Minn.

Olsten Corporation. 1996. Cigna HealthCare selects Olsten Kimberly QualityCare as national provider of home health care services. Unpublished internal news release. February 5.

Olsten Kimberly QualityCare. 1996a. *Network: a publication for Olsten Kimberly QualityCare.* February.

———1996b. *Mission & vision.* Melville, New York. February.

Sprenger, Gordon. 1995. Interview with Ken Jennings. Minneapolis, Minn.

Vision 2000 focus: patients, priorities, programs. 1994. Unpublished report. MetroHealth System.

White, Terry. 1995. Interview with Ken Jennings.

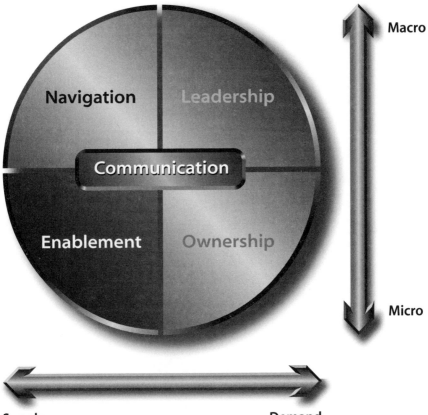

# 10

## ENABLEMENT

As the sea plane approached the sandbar, four Med-Care Plus employees congratulated one another on having come so far. After two days of travel, they had reached the remote Yukon River site. Indianapolis, Indiana and MedCare Plus International, the imaginary employer of the hypothetical quartet in the illustrative story that follows, seemed a million miles away.

Surrounded by tundra, alder, and salmon-filled waters, the four employees alighted from the plane and clambered onto the sandbar. The pilot tossed out a large float with fishing gear, waders, a compass, some rudimentary cooking utensils, and enough mosquito repellent to last them for 15 hours. Then, with a thumbs up, he gunned the plane's engine and roared off, leaving them until 9 p.m., when he would return to take them back to the lodge.

The group—a manager in MedCare Plus' cardiovascular

unit, two home health care experts, and a medical technology specialist—is similar to some twenty others from the managerial ranks of MedCare Plus International, a leader in hospital supplies and managed care. The group's members had all participated in the company's Institute for Training and Development, which provides an intensive curriculum for employees seeking to hone their leadership skills. Dr. David M. Dixon, who directs the Institute for Training and Development, and Dr. Marilyn Powers, who is responsible for organizational effectiveness, see such expeditions as a kind of enablement training and development that helps make the strategy of MedCare Plus happen and makes the business initiatives work.

Robert Adams is MedCare Plus's executive vice president and the CEO of ManageCare Corporation, the health care products and cost-management services company that MedCare Plus International was planning to spin off during the second half of 1996. With sales approaching $5 billion, ManageCare will be the industry leader, employing 20,000 worldwide. Adams believes that the Yukon River adventure provides important training for future leaders of ManageCare. The teamwork and survival skills acquired during the expedition are transferable to the world of health care. The MedCare groups face the challenges of that remote region with enough supplies—except food and water—to survive. Their job is to discover how to use their gear to keep themselves alive.

There was design in that madness. In effect, the four MedCare Plus managers go to learn what many top industry leaders have begun to realize: Identifying the best leaders and instilling a sense of ownership is only half of the change management process. To be successful, health care enterprises must enable their people, processes, and systems to work at peak performance.

As Terry Neill of Andersen Consulting observes, managers need to change their thinking about enabling human resources: Personnel is not so much a resource as a business asset that "deserves at least as sound an investment strategy as [the] company's spending on financial and physical capital." In fact, it is more accurate to use the term human capital rather than the less precise and outdated term "human resources." (Neill 1995: 13)

Given the benefits the company realizes when its people return to Indianapolis, MedCare Plus International considers it a small investment to transport its managers to the remote regions of the Yukon River. Back in Indiana, other MedCare Plus employees enroll in the Institute for Training and Development. They learn to take advantage of the most effective clinical and administrative processes, the most user-friendly systems, and the most productive policies for personnel. Those programs for human-capital development help make the health care organization stronger and better able to drive the change process. Clearly, enablement is a crucial aspect of the transformation journey.

Simply put, enablement includes all the gears, wheels, and springs that make the new health care organization's clock tick: It gives people the tools and the power to get their jobs done well. In this chapter, we look at four key imperatives for today's health care organization:

▼ Design the most effective processes

▼ Create the best design of organizational structures

▼ Promote the creation and sharing of knowledge

▼ Manage performance and professional intellect

Our extensive interviews with health care executives around the world indicate that to get everyone contributing productively, leaders undertaking organizational transformations must work to create significant, sustainable changes in each of those four areas.

### Design the Most Effective Processes

A process defines the way work gets done. Think of a process as a series of interrelated activities designed to produce outcomes for customers or markets. Whatever their products or markets, progressive health care companies are always alert for ways to eliminate non-value-adding processes, improve efficiency, and capitalize on emerging technologies. And whatever the name we give to this activity—work redesign, reengineering, process improvement—the central intention is to change the way organizations do business.

Consider the following examples of creating effective processes that help build the capabilities described in the earlier chapters.

▼ *Emory University Health Communications Project, Atlanta, Georgia:* Technology experts at the project have developed a portable video-broadcast system, nicknamed Picasso, that allows paramedics to send pictures of victims' injuries directly to the university hospital's emergency room. Examining patients even before they arrive, emergency room physicians can now check patients' records and prepare treatments before the ambulance arrives at the hospital. According to Dr. Stephen Holbrook of the university's emergency medical division, "paramedics equipped with Picasso become people who make house calls."

▼ *Nacogdoches Medical Center Hospital, Texas:* When the operating room supervisor at the hospital noticed that each of the six resident surgeons had idiosyncratic supply preferences and consistently ordered certain postsurgical treatments for their patients, she brought this matter to the surgeons' attention. Made aware of escalating costs, the surgeons collaborated and eliminated eighty-three of the 278 steps of such routine procedures as hip-replacement surgery. The redesigned process has cut the hospital's cost for replacement surgery by $3,000 and has reduced the patient's stay from eight to just over four days. (Sasenick 1994: 20)

▼ *Washoe Health System, Reno, Nevada:* When hospital officials recognized the need to reinvigorate the enterprise with state-of-the-art electronic equipment, they established partnerships with vendors to develop diagnostic testing, along with processes for intensive care, medical record maintenance, and inventory control. Granting the vendors the right to sell those processes to other institutions, Washoe can now mount projects that it otherwise could not have afforded.

▼ *Astra Merck:* The most effective processes are typically those fully integrated with the latest innovations in information technology. Cheryl Rothwell, executive director, Licensing and Business Development, and a member of the company's pharmaceutical solutions management team, notes that when planning the new pharmaceutical enterprise, the management team considered using Merck's Corporate Licensing Information System, a huge database originally developed by Merck using Wang technology. That system, however, required as many as forty full-time staff to operate and maintain it. Furthermore, to make use of the data on the some 10,000 compounds in that database, people depended on its operators, who became known for their nearly infallible memories. Whenever staff left, they took valuable access to a storehouse of information.

Weighing those concerns, Astra Merck leaders opted to introduce a more practical system that gives drug developers better access to specific information—for example, which drugs are particularly effective against inflammatory bowel disease—about pharmaceutical products. Moreover, the technology allows them to synthesize the work of independent experts who participate in the development and testing of drugs. (Schön and Moore 1994: 10)

These examples speak to the power of information technology to enable care givers to focus on the patient. Many health care organizations have successfully incorporated such processes while undertaking extensive change programs. At Kaiser Permanente Northern California Region, for example, information technology has created new value for customers, according to Executive Vice President and Regional Manager David Pockell. (Pockell 1995)

Not every new process, of course, has such remarkable effects. Some add little or no value to the organization, while often introducing obstacles of their own to the pursuit of the enterprise's goals. Terry White of MetroHealth Systems, for example, recounts that in the initial stages of a change process, physicians in the ambulatory care area requested a quick-fix solution to the broken phone system. While a fairly straightforward, stopgap measure could have been devised, White and the change management team recognized that without proper connections to other areas at MetroHealth, a temporary solution was no solution. The real answer demanded a cross-functional process, which eventually forced the complete redesign of the ambulatory care program. (White 1995)

When contemplating the difficulties of managing a transformation process, many would-be leaders fear throwing the entire organization into chaos. Better to leave the old system intact, they reason, than to replace dysfunction with disorder. As we have seen, however, true leaders take a much larger view and refuse to equate change with chaos. As part of their overall vision, they see opportunity in the midst of risk. They delight in the chance to make organizational processes efficient and enable employees to work at their most productive level.

## *Create the Best Design of Organizational Structures*

Effective organizational structures are those that free people to do their best work, enabling them to function smoothly in the processes of the organization. The reengineering efforts of the 1980s and 1990s pointed an accusing finger at the inefficiency of multiple managerial levels. Hierarchies are fine for totalitarian governments, but they are essentially unproductive for the complex process redesign and flexible organizations of today.

Furthermore, as we all know, hierarchies are expensive. Generally speaking, the flatter the corporate structures, the more efficient their processes. Lateral structures work best because they encourage everyone to develop a greater sense of ownership and responsibility for the work their teams do. As Larry Bossidy, the CEO of Allied Signal, says, "Hierarchy and authoritarian structures don't involve as many people, so employees don't buy in. And, therefore, they tend to be less successful." (Welch et al. 1993)

Frank LaFasto, vice president of organization effectiveness and development for Baxter Healthcare Corporation, has made a thorough study of team-based design. Based on their analysis of more than 500 teams worldwide, LaFasto and Carl E. Larson, professor of speech communication at the University of Denver, discussed the formation of effective teams in their book *Teamwork: What Must Go Right/What Can Go Wrong*

(1989). When we talked with him, he spoke frankly not only about his personal fight with cancer, which gave him even deeper insights into how health care teams work, but also about his observations on people committing themselves to projects they believe in and value. At Baxter, those values are translated into the organization's "Three Rs," which all teams put at the top of their agendas: Respect, Responsiveness, Results. (LaFasto 1995) With respect for each other and one another's work, team members collaborate more effectively. In other words, LaFasto explains, "Teamwork succeeds most dramatically when team members are enthusiastically unified in pursuit of a common objective rather than individual agendas." (LaFasto and Larson 1989: 84) When the organization inspires true team effort, employees enthusiastically accept the challenges of the transformation.

The leaders of Olsten Kimberly QualityCare know very well how employee buy-in can remove barriers to a change program. In 1996, Olsten Kimberly made the transition from a primarily hierarchical structure to a team-based structure. It sought to inspire a culture dedicated to achieving high performance and the best care for its customers. The results have been outstanding. The Network Development Team, for example, has assembled people with cross-functional responsibilities for specialized patient services across a broad continuum of health care. Olsten Kimberly has set its sights on leading the industry in the delivery of managed care, integrated services, information services, customer consultation, and other areas of health care. According to Joe Mann, a member of the Network Development Team, "the whole is indeed greater than the sum of its parts . . . because the team structure focuses the group's natural competitive forces on achieving strategic goals—with greater results than we could reach on our own." (Olsten 1996a: 7)

Other health care leaders have discovered the benefits of creating a more lateral structure in their organizations. Gail Warden, the CEO of Henry Ford Health System in Detroit, for example, observes that many health care organizations face the problem of retaining good physicians. It is important to offer them sufficient incentives to buy into the corporate structure instead of jumping ship. Monetary compensation is not always enough to accomplish this goal. "You have to make physicians believe and live the idea that they are truly a part of the organization," says Warden, who has spent eight years directing the course of Henry Ford Health System. "Physicians have to sit on the board of directors; they must be involved in making decisions that affect the business aspects of the organization, and they have to believe that they can influence what direction the enterprise takes." (Warden 1995)

Henry Ford Health System has developed a network of independent physicians in some of Detroit's older managed community hospitals. It chose areas of the city where Henry Ford Health System had not already established a commanding presence. Little by little, the organization enlisted the services of physicians who began to develop a sense of collaboration and cooperation rather than head-to-head competition. (Warden 1995) That strategy has helped Henry Ford Health System become a leader in promoting health throughout the community: It moved Henry Ford beyond those segments where private practice was the dominant form of health care and where attention had focused on curing diseases rather than preventing their occurrence in the first place.

For the patient revenue project at Kaiser Permanente Southern California Region, there is a specific team whose focus is to ensure the change process stays on track once the team has moved on. This team identifies those people in the organization who resist the changes and invites them to share their fears in an informal setting. The team members seek to engage their participation by assuring them that their concerns are important. For example, when organizations such as Kaiser Permanente create new processes, some employees move out of traditional functions like billing or admissions. Managers of those departments often feel anger and frustration at losing control. The Kaiser change management team recommends the formation of "infrastructure teams" that bring together people from human resources, public affairs, labor relations, personnel, as well as department administrators. Those teams ensure that changes are made as smoothly as possible, incentives are consistent with business outcomes, and jobs are designed to make the most of employees' skills and knowledge.

The redesign of jobs and management structures requires leaders who truly trust their employees. Whenever there are changes in decision-making authority, people understandably feel as if everything they have grown used to has been uprooted. Their fear manifests itself in emotions ranging from anger and resentment to sheer panic, but with coaching and sustained visioning, effective leaders can design organizational structures that make the best use of human capital.

### Promote the Creation and Sharing of Knowledge

Peter Drucker writes that the "basic economic resource . . . is no longer capital, nor natural resources . . . nor labor. It is and will be knowledge. . . . The *economic* challenge of the post-capitalist society will therefore be the productivity of knowledge work and the knowledge worker." (Drucker 1994)

When asked what attributes the best employees will bring to the future health care enterprise, the industry leaders we interviewed told us knowledge, clear reasoning, and adaptability. To survive in the increasingly competitive health care markets, people will need more than highly developed skills, such as a mastery of the latest surgical procedures and familiarity with high-tech intensive care monitors. They will need to know also how to create, assess, and use the new knowledge the health care industry now demands.

Today's job descriptions, for example, are likely to call for multiskilled people, those who can adapt quickly to new technology, learn new ways of performing tasks or doing business, and create new knowledge. Every industry faces the challenge of capturing and appropriating knowledge. In the information age, those who generate and share knowledge have a much higher chance of survival than those who merely repackage old ideas.

Broadly speaking, the creation and sharing of new knowledge is the hallmark of the fully enabled organization and is central to the successfully transformed enterprise.

As work in health care becomes more complicated and as hierarchical structures give way to lateral organizations, all employees will need retraining and retooling. To ensure quality and consistency, many organizations will turn to multimedia instruction and business simulation to provide hands-on means to acquire new skills and knowledge. The University of Georgia in conjunction with the Medical College of Georgia has developed a model that quite precisely simulates the human eye. Surgical students use it to get the feel for how much pressure to exert in delicate procedures. An essential aspect of successful surgical technique resides in this feel. That new approach provides students with a near-real experience and the opportunity to experiment without the inherent risks of actual ophthalmic surgery.

According to our friend Reinhard Ziegler, managing partner, Performance Design and Development, with Andersen

Consulting, nearly 80 percent of the Fortune 500 companies are using multimedia training for their employees. Just as companies look to JIT (just-in-time) inventory management to help control production costs, they are now thinking in terms of JIT training: Employees will engage in interactive multimedia education whenever the need for new skills arises. Jeff Howell, the director of technology services for Andersen's Worldwide Center for Professional Education in St. Charles, Illinois, says that "we're able to do things with interactive multimedia we couldn't do before. We're able to simulate a client environment so people feel like they're actually working with a client. The net result is that people have deeper competencies, more skills, and knowledge." (qtd. in Marx 1995)

JIT multimedia training will prove especially beneficial in the health care industry with its staggeringly fast rate of advancing technology, knowledge, and the need for new skills. In the 1950s an auto mechanic could handle nearly any repair by referring to a 500-page manual. Today, that manual is more likely to be 500,000 pages long. (Filipczak 1994) With so many new discoveries in diseases, therapies, and treatments, those employees who know how to find, interpret, and apply relevant information will become a health care organization's most valuable contributors.

### Manage Performance and Professional Intellect

Managers of human capital continually ask the vexing questions: What is performance? How can we measure it? It is easy enough to track the performance of a person who produces fifty widgets a day. There is no comparable system, however, to measure the contribution of the person whose idea for the widget put the company in business.

Such issues are immensely complicated in the health care industry. How does one recognize and reward the work of the nurse who devotes extra time to a patient whose health is precariously balanced? Should we compare the performance of the surgeon who performs two open-heart surgeries a day with the work of another surgeon who devotes half of her workday to research and development of a new heart valve? Granted, many outcomes are quantifiable, but just as many cannot be measured by any instruments we now have.

On finding it too difficult to establish objective criteria for evaluation and rewards, some organizations simply give everyone the same cost-of-living raise. To practically no one's satisfaction, heath care has often taken this path. The enterprise of the future, however, cannot afford to rely on traditional measures of evaluation and compensation: An enterprise that undertakes to change its organizational structures and increase profitability needs to manage performance and professional intellect.

We define performance management as the process for understanding, assessing, and rewarding employee performance through explicit measures that specify goals, objectives, and standards. Performance management includes four main principles.

▼ Employees must understand what everyone expects of them and how their work contributes to the success of the organization.

▼ They must understand and agree with the ways in which their performance will be measured and evaluated.

▼ They must receive accurate, timely, and relevant responses to their work so that they know what they are doing well and what they need to improve.

▼ They must see the connection between their performance and the rewards—both financial and nonfinancial—they receive.

The case of St. Ann's Hospital in Columbus, Ohio, presents a clear picture of those four principles. Like most large community hospitals in the United States, St. Ann's needed to undergo significant changes to align its processes and human capital with the changes its leaders wanted to implement. Prior to the change project, for example, the hospital had two independent systems—one for measuring performance, another for rewarding it. In addition, numerous organization-wide programs took responsibility for training employees, developing and keeping track of skills, assigning people to certain jobs, negotiating benefits and rewards, communicating with the staff, and so on. To the practiced eye of an outside evaluator, the system appeared fragmented and hopelessly inadequate to deal with the complexities of human capital.

In fact, it was. St. Ann's scheduled all employees below the level of department director for performance evaluations on the anniversary of their date of hire. The immediate supervisor or department head conducted the evaluations, a theoretically manageable responsibility because of St. Ann's excessively vertical organizational structure. Despite the low ratio of managers to staff (1:15), some managers complained that they did not have the time to complete evaluations. Others simply informed their employees what their annual raises would be; still others shirked responsibility altogether. Caught in this tangled web of manager-employee relations, the Human Resources Department at St. Ann's could not compare evaluations or integrate performance outcomes with compensation plans, corrective discipline, and staff training.

Each year the hospital handed out service awards recognizing the length of service. Like so many other organizations, St. Ann's found this criterion easy to measure—much easier than assessing actual accomplishments, breakthrough discoveries, and quality performance. Rewards based entirely on years of service, however, undermined St. Ann's change program, which aimed to recognize improvements, accomplishments, and best practices at any level.

As the new St. Ann's implemented its change program, it flattened the organizational structure dramatically. The ratio of managers to staff shot up to 1:100, a change that, in effect, ruled out the possibility of investing total authority for evaluating employees' performance in a single person.

St. Ann's instituted, therefore, a multirater appraisal program that asked up to five individuals familiar with an employee's work to contribute to that employee's evaluation. St. Ann's designed the new system to reflect six major criteria:

▼ It must be easy to administer.

▼ It must have clear goals and measures related
  to Key Performance Indicators.

▼ It should be a positive motivator.

▼ It should differentiate performance.

▼ It should provide adequate feedback.

▼ It should be integrated with such systems as compensation, corrective discipline, and training and development.

The insistence on positive motivation reflects employees' long-standing dissatisfaction with traditional appraisals in which an evaluator identifies only faults and shortcomings. Recognizing that its old system produced anxiety and fear of failure, the change management team at St. Ann's insisted that the evaluation incorporate a support-for-success aspect. Aligning programs to recognize and reward creativity, development of new skills, and contributions to the overall organization, the support-for-success system outlined not only what the hospital expected of its employees but also what incentives employees could earn when their performance exceeded minimum standards. St. Ann's provides an excellent example of a health care organization's attempt to recognize, manage, and reward professional intellect.

In their seminal article for *Harvard Business Review,* James Brian Quinn, Philip Anderson, and Sydney Finkelstein propose four levels of professional intellect, the body of knowledge that any professional must command and continue to update.

▼ Cognitive knowledge, which comes through education, certification, and training—the know-what of the discipline.

▼ Advanced skills, or know-how, which apply that learning to real-world situations.

▼ Systems understanding, which the authors call know-why, the deeper knowledge of "cause-and-effect relationships underlying a discipline."

▼ Self-motivated creativity, the ability to "adapt aggressively to changing external conditions and particularly to innovations that obsolesce . . . earlier skills." (Quinn, Anderson, and Finkelstein 1996: 72)

As part of its creation of a new business venture, Astra Merck, Inc., has instituted a performance management system that recognizes the importance of those types of knowledge. Specifically, the company aligned compensation and rewards with career management, training, and recruitment. Astra Merck now constructs a history for an individual's performance, identifying strengths and weaknesses, past and present contributions to the company's success, and potential areas where an employee could provide valuable insight. Once it establishes those parameters, the company selects employees for special training aimed specifically at helping them work more efficiently in teams, develop additional skills, and discover new areas of expertise that support the company's perceptions of its future needs.

Midway through the transformation process at Astra Merck, Matthew Emmens, vice president of marketing and sales, recognized that drug sales of the new venture might not be strong enough to ensure its survival. He and other executives decided to hire and train 500 new sales reps immediately—a daunting task for any enterprise, new or old. Emmens invited those new recruits to a training session at Disney World in Orlando, Florida, where professional actors performed a play that poked fun at the traditional sales pitch of groveling and pushiness. Inspired by the play's projection of a cooperative relationship between salesperson and customer, the 500 new recruits learned to approach clients with information that described how Astra Merck could help improve communications with patients. Today, Astra Merck salespeople become CPR instructors and help train physicians' staffs, and they provide special materials that health care professionals use to educate patients about hypertension. (Schon and Moore 1994: 12–13)

Wayne Yetter, the CEO of Astra Merck, believes that the key to achieving employee buy-in and commitment to the change project is trust. "At Astra Merck, TRUST stands for Truth, Responsibility, Unity, Support, and Teamwork. It's simple," Yetter says, "but it stands for the way we treat one another and for the way we do business with our customers." (LBA Consulting 1995) The hiring and training of 500 new people might send the typical human resources department into apoplectic fits, but Astra Merck leaders recognized in this challenge a way to inspire young recruits and meet customers' demands simultaneously.

Similar challenges confronted the leaders of Aetna Health Plans, who sought to move the company's focus from traditional indemnity to managed care. After identifying Aetna's eight core competencies, executives began reconfiguring job descriptions and realigning the best people across business groups. David Lungrin, vice president for human resources, believes that a key to the success of that management process has been the collection of both employee and customer surveys that provide empirical evidence of success. Moreover, assessment of performance is not a one-way street at Aetna: By answering a dozen or so questions that appear on their computer screens, employees will be able to assess their supervisors and the company itself. Every month, the company compiles and distributes the results of those surveys to supervisors and corporate executives, who regularly monitor the pulse of the enterprise itself.

Although some 5,000 miles separate that sandbar on the Yukon River from Indianapolis, Indiana, those four MedCare Plus employees recognized the power of their new knowledge about themselves and their ability to work as a team. The pilot of the seaplane had left them with the tools they needed to survive, but it was up to them to discover how to don waders, jiggle lures, and dodge low-flying mosquitoes. They earned simple but meaningful rewards: a pan of fresh fish; plenty of clear, clean air; and a heightened sense of their own self-esteem. What's more, they returned to Indiana with a commitment to the success of their team and their organization that would last them throughout their careers. MedCare Plus enabled these people to do a job, and they proved that they could succeed.

# REFERENCES

Drucker, Peter. 1994. *Post-capitalist Society*. Harper Collins.

Filipczak, Bob. 1994. Looking past the numbers. *Training* 31.10 (October): 67–74.

LaFasto, Frank M. J., and Carl E. Larson. 1989. *Teamwork: what must go right/what can go wrong*. Newbury Park: Sage Publications.

———1995. Interview with Ken Jennings.

LBA Consulting Group. 1995. Growth through acquisition. *The Change Manager*, Winter.

Marx, Wendy. 1995. The new high-tech training. *Management Review* 84.2 (February): 57–60.

Neill, Terry. 1995. The critical mindset in strategic change. HR Consulting Tools Conference, Orlando, Fl., December 5.

Olsten Kimberly QualityCare. 1996a. *Network: A Publication for Olsten Kimberly QualityCare Employees*. February: 2–8.

Olsten Kimberly QualityCare. 1996b. Aetna Health Plans sign national home care contract. PRNewswire, Burlington, MA. February 1.

Pockell, David. 1995. Interview with Kurt Miller. October 31.

Quinn, James Brian, Philip Anderson, and Sydney Finkelstein. 1996. Managing professional intellect: making the most of the best. *Harvard Business Review*, March–April, 71–80.

Sasenick, Susan M. 1994. Surgeons spearhead cost-cutting. *Healthcare Forum*, July–August, 20.

Schön, Donald A., and Gwendolyn B. Moore. 1994. *A case study of the Astra Merck engagement: extracting lessons from successes and dilemmas*. Internal case study. Andersen Consulting. September.

Warden, Gail. 1995. Interview with Ken Jennings. November 20.

Welch, John F., Lawrence Bossidy, William Weiss, Michael Walsh, Stratford Sherman, and Joyce E. Davis. 1993. A master class in radical change. *Fortune*, December 13, 82.

White, Terry. 1995. Interview with Ken Jennings.

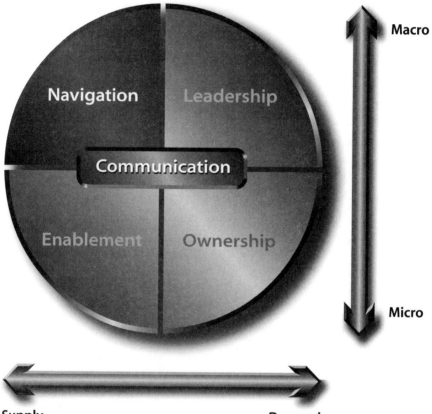

# 11

## NAVIGATION

W hen Kathryn Stevens of Kaiser Permanente's Southern California Region requested permission to hire a cultural anthropologist, few of her colleagues grasped the reason. A cultural anthropologist? But Stevens, the project leader of Kaiser's effort to reengineer the way medical offices and hospitals collect for their services, had an explanation for the doubters: The anthropologist's perspective enhances team members' understanding of how best to implement and sustain improved processes amidst cultural change. (Stevens 1995)

Guiding change is the essence of Stevens' job. Kaiser Permanente senior management has charged her with making sure that receptionists, billers, financial counselors, physicians, and other staff members collect accurate health plan eligibility information, counsel patients on how various health care coverages apply to them, and quickly bill patients and their insurers for amounts due. Because Kaiser had not captured all needed information in the past, the organization had forgone a great deal of revenue. With the improved identification process, the Southern California region will obtain the needed data as soon as patients enter the care delivery system. The process will bring an estimated $25 million more revenue each year from sources such as private insurers and government-funded programs.

The conversion to the new process, however, takes time as well as persistence because it means a change in the organizational unit's culture. "The problem we have had is that we have made lots of wonderful incremental improvements," explains Stevens, "but they often unraveled soon after the change management team members were gone." (Stevens 1995)

Some of the unraveling stems from overburdening medical office and emergency department staff with the work of installing new processes while they struggle to keep up with day-to-day business. In busy clinics, during flu season, with a stream of people flooding through the doors of doctors' offices, the new process goes out the window. This is understandably so, too. The process calls for receptionists to ask patients a number of questions and, when push comes to shove, to ignore the process to put the needs of the patient first. (Benson 1995)

But much of the unraveling comes from people reverting to old habits, beliefs, and behaviors. The challenge for Stevens and similar change leaders, then, is how to create permanent change when people at Kaiser Permanente, like those in any organization, tend to revert to the status quo. The organization solved this problem in part by hiring cultural anthropologist Judith Benson as a member of the change management team to examine the Kaiser Permanente culture. The team could then observe the cultural barriers that would block the assimilation of change. (Stevens 1995)

Assessing current organizational culture is one of the first steps all organizations must take as they prepare to navigate through all the changes such a journey requires. Navigation, the fourth quadrant of journey management, has the following three phases.

▼ *Assessing the context of change:* Thoroughly understanding change drivers, stakeholder expectations, readiness for change, and organizational culture, politics, technology, and strategy.

▼ *Planning the change journey:* Developing change programs, phases, timelines, performance measures, and reporting.

▼ *Managing the change journey:* Coordinating and integrating change initiatives, analyzing and reporting on performance, and adjusting program management accordingly. ("Manage" 1995)

Robert A. Lauer believes that managers who guide change according to the principles of navigation can assure that the change is well planned, delivered, monitored, and measured, and that duplication of effort or programs is minimized. (Lauer 1996) Additionally, they avoid launching a slate of initiatives that conflict with each other or overburden the organization with too much change all at once. Managers must also understand the organization's capacity to change and how to create this capacity and apply it to the proper initiative. This requires identification and alignment of many attributes—such as leadership, the change processes, and culture. (Lauer 1996)

Organizations that do not use change navigation techniques will fail to reach targets on time, waste money and energy fighting avoidable conflicts between stakeholders, and undercut employee and investor confidence in management. Those who do follow the techniques of navigation will find that they can better prioritize change projects based on payback, carry out multiple overlapping changes while continuing to operate successfully, ensure that change initiatives complement each other, manage the pacing of change initiatives so they come on stream only at the rate the organization can absorb, and deliver maximum benefits with minimum cost, effort, and disruption.

Many health care companies regard conflict, false starts, and confusion as the price management must pay when changing direction or goals. But these companies can achieve effective change when leaders apply hard disciplines to planning and management of changes in people, processes, and technology.

### Assessing the Context

The first of the three phases of navigation is assessing the context. Even if executives and managers of change have a good idea of where they want to lead the organization, they may have a much poorer idea than they thought of where the organization is coming from. Any program to manage change must begin with understanding the status quo. Managers cannot know how to remold the organizational form if they are in the dark about the form they are starting with.

Getting a sharp picture of that form comes from assessing a variety of factors that make up the organizational context. The first step in clarifying the context is analyzing stakeholders, decision makers, and others who have influence in the direction the organization needs to take. For the patient revenue reengineering project at Kaiser Permanente Southern California, this task fell to the assessment team, which in January

1995 began by interviewing the executives on the region's project steering committee, as well as midlevel administrators and managers in charge of the revenue collection process. "What we really tried to do is get to the people who were respected throughout the organization, whose judgments and opinions were highly valued," says Judith Benson. (Benson 1995)

The team sought to find out what each person thought the project would achieve. They also asked for people's views on the strengths and weaknesses of the current systems. They even held focus groups with the middle managers to confirm what senior management was saying. "We really wanted to know what we were going to get into," Benson says. "Where were our land mines? We wanted to identify them up front." (Benson 1995) The interviews also helped the team identify potential resisters, including those who might feign support for the change but later fight behind the scenes to retain old processes.

Organizations undergoing change must thoroughly understand the context of their cultures. Here again, the project sponsors at Kaiser Permanente relied on the change management team to expose the written and unwritten tenets of its culture. For example, team members were aware that the Kaiser culture understandably called on people to focus above all else on patient care. According to Benson, "The dollars that came in to support patient care were not a primary concern." People simply didn't value the handling of money matters. That showed that the change program would have to stress the maintenance of quality of care while it focused people's attention on collecting the money Kaiser Permanente was due for its services. (Benson 1995)

The project team's work also contributed to a third task in assessing the context of change: evaluating the organization's capability for change. ("Manage the Journey" 1995) Every organization must get answers to some hard questions: Are people knowledgeable about change itself? Have their jobs stressed learning and continuous change to improve work and processes? Are people personally predisposed to tackling projects with uncertain outcomes? How have previous change journeys worked out? What did the organization learn?

Like managers in many other organizations, the change team encountered a strong "not invented here" attitude within Kaiser Permanente. The people running revenue collection processes in medical offices and hospitals and other administrative units often doubted the team could design a standard process that would work in their local area. (Stevens 1995) The change program would thus have to deal with high levels of skepticism.

Another task in assessing the context of change is analyzing the environment—the factors inside and outside the organization that affect the management of change. As managers prepare for change, they must understand internal issues of technology, politics, strategy, the priority of competing initiatives, the budgeting of time and money, and so on. They must also understand external issues, such as falling technology costs, new technological capabilities, economic cycles, social trends, and the changing winds of politics and regulation.

Included in this analysis must be a look at the specific drivers of change and how they may affect the change program. Kaiser Permanente, for example, was reacting to the emergence of a huge and growing stream of revenues from non-dues-paying patients. This stream had several sources. As employers shifted more of the burden of paying for health care to their employees, Kaiser was starting to receive more revenue as copayments and payments for carve-out services. As payers have started to limit their contributions for care, revenues have come increasingly from Medicare and California's

MediCal payments. As health care competition has continued to heat up in California, fresh revenue has come from patients who freely choose Kaiser Permanente services and products. The upshot for Kaiser has been that, between 1989 and 1993, revenue from non-dues-paying patients jumped from $635 million to $1.9 billion, a 30 percent average annual compound growth rate. (Abbott et al. 1995)

Not only was Kaiser Permanente not getting bills out to all non-dues-paying patients, its complicated revenue collection work flow could add a staggering 500 days to the average life of a patient bill. (Abbott et al. 1995) An analysis of change drivers showed indisputably that Kaiser Permanente had to figure out a better way to manage revenue collection, "to capture the right information, bill the right party the right amount, and collect the money right away." ("Manage the Journey" 1995)

The final task in assessing the context is building a business case. Once managers fully understand the current organization and its environment, they synthesize their assessment to create a compelling story for the necessity for change. That then becomes an essential ingredient for both the second stage in navigation and for leaders building buy-in throughout the organization.

## Planning the Change Journey

The second phase of change navigation is planning the journey so people, processes, and technology all work together smoothly. Planning change, like planning life, can make all the difference in how fast and smoothly organizations transform themselves. As writer William DeMille once wrote, "We are all pilgrims on the same journey . . . but some pilgrims have better maps." The planning phase of navigation provides a clear map of the organization's origin, travel route, and change destination.

This element of planning is to create a from-to summary. The summary juxtaposes the current context with the sought-after future. A good example of a summary of the future was put together by Olsten Kimberly QualityCare. Its road map, discussed briefly in Chapters 9 and 10, specifies shared values, new behaviors, and key elements of the vision, such as delivering managed care, integrating services for customers, and adopting the Gold Standard, the company's set of reengineered administrative processes. Olsten Kimberly QualityCare employees have posted this road map in the company's 600 branches to remind them where they are headed.

The second element of change journey planning is a detailed plotting of the organizational change program. This plan must clearly specify every change initiative, event, and milestone. It should give snapshots of the business architecture at a series of important steps along the journey of change. And it should specify the pace of change, matched to expectations, change readiness, and other limitations revealed during the assessment phase.

As a part of this planning, managers should pay special attention to the opportunity for quick wins. Where can the organization make changes—early and easily—that will enliven employee interest in change? Where can the organization get a big benefit, fast? Olsten Kimberly QualityCare's president, Robert Fusco, acknowledges that he set expectations high: the redesign of the entire organization, the reengineering of all branches according to the Gold Standard, the revolution of corporate culture, and the growing of a brand new managed care business. Still he says, "Common sense tells us that although stretch goals are important, we need to create opportunities for small wins along the way. It's the little victories that create momentum. They fuel our sense of urgency . . . mark our progress and reward us for our hard work." (Fusco 1996a}

Another element of planning is what we call milestone planning: a package of initiatives aimed at implementing a new organizational capability. A change journey comprises one or many milestones for advancing the organization in controlled stages along the path to its destination. Olsten Kimberly QualityCare, for example, did not reach every new capability all at once. Instead, it launched in separate phases the reengineering to standardize branch-office operations, the training to create a new culture that stressed teamwork, and the revamped business capabilities needed to make the company more like a managed care firm. (Fusco 1996b).

The fourth key step in the planning phase of navigation is the creation of a system for performance analysis and reporting. Of foremost importance is that managers clearly state, in measurable terms, what they hope to achieve by undertaking the change. They must then also specify the multiple interim outcomes that, along the way to the change destination, will contribute to the target outcome. If the target is, say, to double productivity, interim targets measure not only productivity improvements to date but also progress in implementing the change initiatives—roadshows, training programs, new technology—that contribute to higher productivity. The targets also measure soft factors, such as changes in behavior, culture, management practices, and attitudes, as evidenced by employee survey data.

The final element in journey planning is to create a communication plan, precisely the same requirement for developing ownership. As explained in Chapter 9, the communication plan is far more than a tool to communicate news; it is itself a vehicle for making the change take hold.

### *Managing the Journey*

The third and final phase of change navigation is managing implementation. Contrary to some executives' thinking, you can't throw a bunch of bright people on a change project and expect the job to get done. The network of change managers needs a disciplined process for micromanaging, far more detailed than for the day-to-day running of the organization. Only constant focus on program management specifics will assure the change program stays on track and on schedule.

The most basic element of journey management is establishing solid, day-to-day management practices. In our experience, that means firmly rooting throughout the organization a set of project management practices in which employees clearly understand the policies, processes, procedures, and tools. Program management then builds from this cultural and managerial common ground.

The crucial element of journey management is the management of the change programs themselves—coordinating initiatives, allocating money and people to projects, and managing schedules. One organization that took a comprehensive approach to managing its journey of change was the finance department of Pfizer, Inc. In 1994, Pfizer set out to reengineer its accounts payable process to become more customer focused, more concentrated on value-added tasks, and increasingly streamlined. To assure the company stayed on track, Pfizer managers created an overall program management plan, along with detailed work plans that specified scores of steps in implementing training, communications, new job profiles, a new organizational structure, new performance measures, and new employee skills. Pfizer calculated how much time each initiative and its many components would take, creating in essence an overall program management map that then structured its management of change every step of the way.

The communication plan created by Pfizer was especially detailed, outlining a year-long schedule of deliverables. For example, Pfizer kicked off the change program by announcing it in its internal finance newsletter. It followed this January 1994 announcement over the next year with fifty additional communication vehicles and events—from memos to fliers to classroom training—each timed to support, strengthen, and further the change program. Pfizer also set forth a list of the tasks for local change agents ("user champions"), specifying their activities month to month. In March 1994, for example, the champions worked with headquarters to define their roles and responsibilities. In May, they compiled feedback on a conference room pilot.

A particularly helpful device during any change program is what many organizations call a war room. This is a conference room dedicated to the change program, a spot where change managers can lay out their battle plans for implementing change and keep track of their release of change initiatives, feedback, and necessary adjustments to future plans. Many organizations we work with paper the walls of these nerve centers with charts and maps, graphically showing the scope of change projects and the progress of each. The war room is also a place where the team can store its archives, methods binders, and other documents.

Another helpful device in journey management is the change contract. The network of change managers will negotiate contracts with a variety of divisions and local units to codify the game plan for change. The prime purpose of the contract is for the change network to secure funding for the change from the many units involved. But the contracts will also detail the mission of the change network, the structure of the network, the obligations of different partners, the methodology the network will use, the schedules and deadlines for the different phases of change, and other details such as quality assurance and monitoring. Because the contracts require formal negotiation and signing, they give a highly visible structure to the details of managing change. They also require everyone involved to think through the change program so that people encounter fewer surprises along the way.

The third element of managing the change journey is monitoring, which includes tracking, analyzing, and reporting performance. In large-scale changes, network managers must build systems to monitor performance at the local, intermediate, and corporate-wide levels. The systems at all three levels should dovetail, so that performance measures or reporting categories at the lowest levels feed higher levels.

Monitoring systems should measure performance of three kinds: business performance, changes in employee attitudes and behaviors, and change-program progress. In other words, network managers must determine, first, whether the change program is on schedule; second, whether people are changing with it; and third, whether the organization is reaping the business benefits desired.

Managers can get this information with the help of a variety of tools, including scorecards, reports, meetings, and electronic bulletin boards. The core monitoring tools, however, are report cards and reports. Each of these tools feeds information to managers of meetings for war-room strategy sessions and for executive review of the overall program. The report cards can track both soft and hard data, although the more quantitative the data the better, making it easier to understand trends and roll the information up to higher levels in aggregate form.

One example of a scorecard is the one used by Pfizer in its accounts payable process. Pfizer chose to use an A through F grading system. A month after it launched its reengineered accounts-payable processes, it created its "month one" report card to figure out if the new processes were working as planned. For example, for performance in handling standard voucher entries, Pfizer gave itself an A ("exceeds expectations"). For performance in meeting its target of one-time voucher entry, it gave itself a C– ("needs significant improvement"). And for the process of handling petty cash, it gave itself a C+. In each case, Pfizer managers could quickly see trouble spots, identify possible solutions, and verify the urgency of proceeding with planned solutions such as creating a new, standardized petty cash form. Not only did the report card give Pfizer managers a performance assessment, it actually helped spur further change by highlighting shortfalls.

As a part of the monitoring system, managers should take care to create the kinds of measures and questions that will allow executives to compare costs with benefits. What is working? What isn't? Is the change journey delivering the goods? Which projects should managers consider canceling? This type of cost-benefit analysis requires that managers find a means to connect the changes to financial gains or losses. Although some change projects aim to improve quality or service, and not cost directly, they still must prove their worth by improving the organization's financial picture in some indirect way.

Once Kaiser Permanente changed over some of its sites to its new revenue collection process, for example, the organization began tracking the increase in the few people that receptionists and financial counselors identified as ineligible for coverage as Kaiser members. Proper identification is the first step in finding alternative sources of payment. Nonmember identification at one site shot up 20 percent. Billings at that site then increased from $290,000 to $430,000 per week. Predictably, after a lag of about three months, Kaiser Permanente's cash flow from alternative billings at that site increased proportionally. Although the organization received a shot in the arm from a one-time backlog reduction of over $500,000, Kaiser Permanente could not have done without a well-managed change program supplemented with careful monitoring.

Altogether, the elements of navigation make the entire change program come together as a coherent whole. Assessing, planning, executing—none of these journey management steps is mysterious, but each receives too little attention. As the health care industry continues to undergo rapid change, navigation will soar in importance. As Leland Kaiser has stated, the industry has entered a permanent period of white water, when change is not the exception, it is the rule. The leaders of the winning health care enterprise must learn the methods and skills to run the processes and train the people while the organization is in constant flux. Otherwise, they put themselves at risk of wandering aimlessly. They will not reap the benefits they seek.

# REFERENCES

Abbott, Craig, et al. 1995. Patient revenue reengineering. Steering committee background report. Unpublished document. March 8.

Benson, Judith. 1995. Interview with Ken Jennings and Sharyn Materna.

Fusco, Robert A. 1996a. Going for the goal: small wins can make a big difference. *Network: a publication for Olsten Kimberly QualityCare employees*, February, 11.

————1996b. Interview with Sharyn Materna, Ken Jennings, and Mike Reynee.

Lauer, Robert A. 1996. Interview with Ken Jennings.

Manage the journey: quality management prompter. 1995. Andersen Consulting. Unpublished report.

Stevens, Kathryn. 1995. Interview with Sharyn Materna.

# PART IV

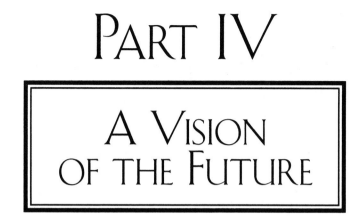

A VISION
OF THE FUTURE

# 12

## CREATING THE FUTURE

James H. Clark, the celebrated founder of Netscape Communications, jumped into the health care business with the help of a bad ankle. As he suffered with a deteriorated, liquefied bone, he hungered to find out every detail about his affliction. That led him to a very simple conclusion that would have far-reaching implications: "For a month there [while I was in pain]," he says, "I would have paid a lot of money to get access to information." (Clark 1996)

A founder not only of Netscape, but of Silicon Graphics, Clark knew plenty about access to information. He saw the lack of information access in health care as a big problem for consumers—painfully so for him. He also saw the promise of using his company's revolutionary Internet browser to solve that problem. So with not more than six months of preparation, Clark launched a new business, Healthscape, now known as Healtheon Corporation, aimed at building a brand new way of handling health care information using his company's world-beating Netscape Navigator software. (Clark 1996; Pitta 1996)

To at least a few blue-sky health care pundits, Clark's new venture was predictable. In fact, at the very same time Clark schemed to create his new company, a group of leading thinkers from the Australian health care community had declared in a report that the two biggest drivers of change in health care would be, first, the transformational use of technology, and second, new entrants into the health care market. (Morlet and Oliver 1995; Oliver, Morlet, and Weerasingam 1995) These seers of the future of the health care industry would not be a bit surprised by the establishment of this new business venture.

But far more significant for managers is that Clark's move wasn't predictable in its particulars; after all, he was not even a participant in the health care industry. He was a one-time Stanford University computer-science professor and a high-tech guru. Health care wasn't his bailiwick. Even today he readily defers to his top managers to explain specifics in the jargon health care managers understand. In short, Clark was a competitor who nobody in health care could easily have singled out before he launched Healtheon.

For that very reason, the creation of Healtheon conveys an important message best heeded by all health care leaders: Some of the biggest change in the future of health care won't come from smooth, incremental evolution. It will come from abrupt, irregular revolution, neither slow nor foreseeable. Industry insiders and outsiders alike will spur this change, as they strive to find new, inventive ways to deliver value to consumers—lower costs, higher quality, better access, more choice, and better service. The lesson for health care managers is that they must forever scan the horizon and position themselves for the unexpected.

## Continuous Change

Clark's story could be taken as a reminder that, as many business writers say, "The only constant is change." But that would be missing the more important message. Clark shows that managers must distinguish between two kinds of change— continuous and discontinuous—and must prepare in different ways for each.

Up to this point, we have focused on the issues of continuous change and the evolution of organizations in the health care industry over the next several years. In the first three parts of this book, we have sketched out the process for organizations to win at continuous change. It requires pursuing our three-part formula: setting new strategies, building competencies to support them, and following the four quadrants of journey management to guide the organizational change.

The story of how Ronald Compton, chairman of Aetna, has reinvented his company in recent years summarizes a number of important points about winning at continuous change. Several years ago, Compton and his management team realized that managed care competitors were eroding Aetna's traditional indemnity business. To satisfy the changing needs of indemnity customers, Aetna brought to market a number of different managed care products. As the market continued to evolve, however, Compton quickly saw that offering managed care services couldn't remain an adjunct to the core indemnity business, it would have to become the core business. Says Compton: "When we looked at what we had, we said, 'Wow, we've got the makings here of a terrific future, but [today] we are largely mainframe oriented, big-customer oriented, and indemnity oriented.'" (Compton 1996b) Aetna didn't have the strategies or competencies to navigate into the managed care future.

After a series of intense strategic planning sessions, Aetna senior managers decided that the company would invest heavily in building its managed care capabilities. It built physicians' networks, rolled out brand-new health plans to employers nationwide, and developed new claims and administrative processes. Still, after a couple of years, Compton believed the company was at risk of becoming a straggler. While it worked quickly to build its competencies and fulfill its strategies, the rapid evolution of the market seemed to outpace the changes in the company. Just three years ago, for example, 65 percent of Aetna's beneficiaries were enrolled in indemnity plans. By the spring of 1996, 65 percent were enrolled in managed care plans. (McGuire 1996)

"As we kept track of what was happening in the outside world, it was clear that we would not [develop a strong form of managed care] in time to really capitalize [on it in the market]," Compton says. "We needed to get to the future faster." (Compton 1996b)

So Aetna senior managers sat down and identified the critical success factors for the company to take the lead in managed care. They also identified the gaps between Aetna's set of competencies and the desired set. The areas of shortfall included managed care management skills, retail selling of managed care products, clinical practice and outcomes management, and geographic market breadth and penetration. (Compton 1996b)

With the analysis in hand, Compton then publicly declared that Aetna wouldn't try to go it alone in propelling itself to national leadership in managed care. Instead, it would rely on an acquisition as the tool to fill out its repertoire of managed care capabilities. While outsiders debated Aetna's moves, Compton and his senior managers spent months scrutinizing some of the biggest names in managed care. In April 1996, Compton announced that Aetna's partner would be

U.S. Healthcare, a much-admired HMO that could help the new Aetna, Inc., bring to market the full complement of strengths that will define excellence in managed care in the years ahead.

"It is an excellent strategic fit," says Compton, who believes that putting the two companies together establishes a strong basis for growth, product innovation, and superior financial performance. (Compton 1996a) Aetna brought to the table a national brand name, diverse product offering, nationwide market penetration, large-scale information-processing capabilities, and long-term relationships with 25 percent of the Fortune 1,000. U.S. Healthcare contributed top-of-the-line skills in managed care administration, cost and quality management, selling directly to consumers, and running advanced systems to track and improve clinical practices and medical outcomes. (Compton 1996a, 1996b) "Combining these strengths," says Compton, "the new enterprise will be positioned to grow rapidly by offering customers a wide variety of products and services on a national scale." (Compton 1996a)

The organization will also be positioned for the rapid and continuous change that all health care organizations face in the next few years. Foremost among the changes is the evolution of organizations from a narrow role of curing disease to a broader one of managing people's health so they don't get sick in the first place. As Compton phrases the immediate challenge: "We really don't have much heath care in this country; we have a lot of sickness cure." But with the U.S. Healthcare acquisition, he says, "We are going to come out of this thing on the other end—managing for health." (Compton 1996b)

As Compton manages for this kind of continuous change, however, he knows from his experience in radically restructuring his company from a traditional insurer to a health care Goliath that he must always prepare for additional uncertainties ahead. Even at the close of the U.S. Healthcare acquisition, he admitted, "This is not the end. . . . We are already thinking about the future of what might come after this." (Compton 1996b)

Trend lines don't extend forever, after all. Sometimes they dissipate, or diverge, or break out in a revolutionary new direction. That means that while managers try to keep up with short-term continuous change, they have to remain equally alert for discontinuous change.

### Discontinuous Change

Discontinuous change can, in a matter of months, turn a high-flying business into a dinosaur. The reason is that discontinuous change can come from so many different and unexpected sources. When the Australian health care experts convened by Andersen Consulting put their heads together, for example, they came up with scores of unknowns that could change the course of the industry. Among them were: socioeconomic forces (such as the displacement of laid-off workers), political pressures (such as the need to provide equity in access), professional-organization pressures (to adjust to new patterns of specialization), economics (national budget deficits), demographic patterns (aging of populations), privatization (of public services), advances in medical technology (such as in noninvasive procedures), and new biotechnology products (genetic research yielding breakthrough treatments). (Oliver, Morlet, and Weerasingam 1995)

In this final chapter, for the sake of illustration, we would like to highlight five potential sources of discontinuous change: the eventual ubiquity of information technology, the growing demystification of medicine, the emerging new consumerism, the migration of health care funding to private sources, and the globalization of health care services. Each of these forces has the clear potential to divert the industry onto an entirely new track.

### *Information Technology*

Information technology has already started to do so. Witness Jim Clark's new start-up. Given that the emerging market for health care data cries out for standards, innovation, and investors' capital, Clark could employ his unique skills and financial wherewithal to shape that market in ways few health care organizations could foresee (and amass a huge share of that market for himself).

Clark's ideas actually hint at a larger, rapidly emerging concept Andersen Consulting calls the Healthcare Infocosm. The Healthcare Infocosm enables individual consumers, providers, and other stakeholders to come together to obtain and provide health information and services in cyberspace. In this technology-enabled world of the future, traditional notions of time, place, and form—which frequently act as barriers or constraints to connecting with the consumer—take on very different meanings. For instance, time becomes irrelevant because every time there is a need, customers can reach out directly to a source of information and knowledge. No longer are they bound by the *hours of operation* of their physicians' office or their health plan's customer-service center.

Distance becomes less relevant because virtually everything can be digitized. Thus, the need for consumers or providers to travel to receive services—most of which are information based—is largely diminished. A nurse advice line with two-way video monitors in Denver can serve a consumer in Vancouver as easily as one located just down the street.

The following scenario would play out many times over: A male patient, new to town, visits his primary care physician and complains of weight loss and coughing. As part of his workup, the physician takes a chest X-ray that reveals enlarged lymph nodes, meaning there is a high chance of tuberculosis. Because TB is so contagious, immediate therapy using three different drugs is needed. The Healthcare Infocosm would enable the physician to immediately access and review the patient's prior medical record and X-rays from his previous physician, to verify that this is a new finding. After confirming this is a new finding, he develops a care plan that is immediately made available to a community health nurse to coordinate a workup and monitor his compliance with the suggested medication regimen. This care plan is also made available to a nutritionist to assist with the necessary dietary counseling.

The gradual capture of pertinent patient data raises the possibility of a future where everyone's medical record and life care plan are essentially portable. In such a world, consumers could authorize the release of their files to the care provider of their choice. They could move from provider to provider and plan to plan, easily followed by their files, getting a checkup from one source, physical therapy from another, and nutrition counseling from still another. The portable patient record and life care plan would assure the continuity of their care.

In the era of the portable patient record, consumers may find the fixed provider networks of managed care organizations particularly confining. They may prefer to create smaller, personalized provider networks of their own, for their market of one, in the same way as consumers of years past. Examples of this already exist in other industries. In the financial services industry, for instance, many individual consumers essentially act as architects of their own financial services system by selecting banks, mutual funds, brokers, and personal financial planners. The ramifications of consumers controlling their own records, and with them the choice of each health care transaction, are hard to predict but will no doubt demand that all health care organizations rethink their business models.

Equally hard to predict are the ramifications of health care professionals having access to all the administrative and clinical information available through the Infocosm. Powered by 21st-century communications technology, the Infocosm will facilitate communication among people and organizations miles apart, rendering it as immediate and personal as if people were working in the same office. This immediacy opens the door to the unbundling of business functions that will make the outsourcing of functions we see today look like managerial baby steps by comparison.

Unbundling allows the functions formerly linked closely in one institution to break apart and work separately. In other words, the people, processes, and data do not have to be physically linked. They can be decoupled and made portable across multiple organizations. Such unbundling will create a future where the competition of organizations and individuals is decided by the value they provide consumers. The strategy of organizations will have to shift even further away from amassing a vertical network of coordinated services. They must migrate instead toward knitting together scores of best-in-class unbundled services within the greater Infocosm. Consumers will likely embrace such a virtual structure since even today they care far less about the organization that serves them than they do about friendly, coordinated service.

## Demystification of Medicine

A second potential source of discontinuous change is the demystification of medicine. By demystification we mean, first, the translation of the complex language and practices of medicine into terms that consumers can easily grasp, and second, the placement of that information within easy reach of consumers. Although the Infocosm will greatly accelerate demystification, technology available today has already opened the gates for its advance. Online databases, multimedia computers, and the Internet offer a cornucopia of new medical advice. As time goes on, however, consumers will probably call for ever greater detail and variety, particularly on care protocols, clinical guidelines, and outcomes research analysis. As consumers digest such information in ever-growing volume, they will continue to recast the roles of players in the health care industry.

One possible consequence is that consumers will supplant physicians as the most powerful influence on health care. Physicians today play basically two roles. They intervene in acute cases to cure what ails their patients, and they dispense advice in nonacute cases. The information spread by the Infocosm is already beginning to reduce their role as advisors in nonacute cases. In some cases, they will be disintermediated by consumers who prefer to go directly to the source of information themselves or to tap into smart software that guides them in their own diagnosis and treatment. This is already happening with individuals who have rare chronic conditions, such as Lou Gherig's disease. Those individuals have formed numerous self-help groups operating through the Internet and in many cases have more comprehensive, up-to-date information on their condition and various treatment options than their own physicians do.

As Tom Ferguson of Harvard Medical School observes, informed consumers will opt first for self-care. They will next turn for advice to friends, family, self-help networks, professional health advisors (such as dial-up nurse practitioners), and particularly the online groups who daily discuss symptoms, treatments, and complications. Only then will they choose to pick up the phone and call the physician. We don't know how this will affect health care in the long term, but the implication is that organizations that focus on filling the growing need will press physicians, clinics, and hospitals to articulate where their services add maximum value and to change their business models accordingly.

## A New Consumerism

The third potential source of discontinuous change is the growth of consumer empowerment and demand. As consumers' appetite for entertainment products has grown with no apparent limit, so will their appetite for health products, defined to include wellness, fitness, nutrition, and related services. Many consumers, especially younger ones, spend heavily on products and services that help them feel better. They are likely to continue to redefine the health care market to include not just a narrow set of products that cure disease, but a much broader set that encompasses everything that helps them live healthier lives. In fact this is happening already. Consumers are voting with their pocketbooks about what constitutes health every day. Last year they spent billions on health-related services outside of traditional insurance premiums and care services. So while most health plans and providers are being continually squeezed on cost, those other organizations tapping into the wants and desires of consumers are generating significant revenues and healthy margins.

Although nobody knows how fast consumer demand for health and health care products will grow, we are confident that the growth will call for organizations to remake themselves to meet the increase. As employer payers squeeze managed care organizations to reduce margins from as high as 30 percent to 8 percent or less, traditional medicine may well become less profitable; thus health care organizations will feel compelled to launch new services. The pattern the health care industry may well follow is the same followed earlier by financial services, where in response to falling margins on basic services such as savings accounts and stock brokerage, companies have introduced a stream of new value-added, higher-margin products.

Some of the products and services traditional organizations will offer include personal health navigation, in which experts explain complex offerings and alternatives and help consumers develop plans and choices for themselves. We also expect a huge expansion of what we today call alternative medicine. Many physicians still look askance at herbal medicine practitioners, chiropractors, meditation instructors, acupuncturists, and the like. But as consumers come to believe that these professionals add real value, organizations will feel compelled to broaden their menu of offerings to please customers and to tap new sources of revenue.

Because of the growing number of opportunities, new entrants are likely to flock to serve the health care market—often from unexpected industries. Software companies like Microsoft will offer online information services and intelligent software. Consumer product companies like Procter & Gamble and General Mills have already created new potions and foods for people with various ailments and risks. Industrial companies such as John Deere & Company have already created wellness and health services of their own. Even entertainment giants like the Walt Disney Company have gotten into the act, offering services (as we shall see later in the chapter) that combine high technology, entertainment, lifestyle enhancement, and traditional health care. Health care managers should prepare themselves for these new entrants, who will create an endless stream of products, services, or bundles of both to sell directly to consumers.

### *Shifts in Financing*

A fourth source of discontinuous change could come from reforms in the way society funds health care. Today, employers and the government pay most of the bills, and they in turn exercise a great deal of control over how the money is spent. But lawmakers continue to introduce proposed legislation to create tax advantages for medical savings accounts. These accounts, whether sponsored by employers, self-employed workers, or by Medicare or Medicaid administrators, would give the consumer direct purchase authority. If that happens, consumers will allocate not only discretionary dollars but also money formerly considered a part of their mandatory, nondiscretionary monthly expenses.

Again, nobody knows how consumers, now holding the purse strings of health care, will spend their money. According to Dr. Bob Blenden of the Harvard School of Public Health, they might buy largely according to the appeal of the benefit plan offered: The more variety and choice for a fixed price, for example, the better the perceived deal. Or perhaps they will buy according to where they get the best service—wherever organizations routinely hire attentive nurses and doctors. Or perhaps they'll take the hard-nosed-buyer approach and purchase services based on outcomes measures that demonstrate which providers deliver the highest quality. (Blenden 1995) All we know for sure is that consumers represent a wild card: They could swing billions of dollars away from some markets and into others.

## Globalization of Health Care

A fifth source of potential discontinuous change is the globalization of health care. In most of the world, organizations that supply hands-on care delivery and health coverage services operate primarily at local or regional levels within individual countries. With few exceptions, such as the limited cross-border activity of large pharmaceutical and medical supply companies—and a small handful of emerging U.S.-based managed care and niche organizations—health care organizations in different countries don't directly compete with each other. But in a world connected by the Infocosm, organizations in different regions, even in different countries, will compete with each other. Companies like United Healthcare and Access Health are already establishing operations outside of the United States. The competition will become especially fierce in the provision of health care information services, where excellence has little dependence on the location of the provider. Such services will include health counseling, intelligent software, even dial-a-doc services. In the same way that product quality allowed Japanese automakers to give U.S. manufacturers a run for their money, health care service quality, coming from whatever source, will give local organizations a run for that part of their business where care giver and care receiver don't have to meet face to face. A cardiologist authorized by a consumer to view health care records online, for example, can dispense a second opinion from anywhere, taking business away from local practitioners.

These five sources of potential discontinuous change, to say nothing of the scores of others that could burst onto the scene, argue that discontinuous change warrants constant consideration. They also show why making mistakes in positioning the organization for the future is so easy: Anticipating the future is devilishly hard. Managing change based on such predictions is even more difficult because organizations have trouble giving credence to any view of the future that flies in the face of shared visions and assumptions that, although now obsolete, have helped make those organizations successful.

The health care industry today, for example, is founded on several assumptions that may well be candidates for the boneyard. One of them is that medical knowledge resides with a few highly trained people, mainly physicians. Another is that all health services are delivered by licensed care givers in dedicated buildings. A third is that health care is a local or regional business. A fourth is that employers or governments are the primary sources of health care funding. As we have seen, these assumptions make a shaky foundation for building visions of the health care future. Health care managers intent on keeping their organizations positioned for discontinuous change must regularly challenge such long-held beliefs.

## A Vision of the Future

One organization that is leading the way in positioning itself for discontinuous change is Celebration Health, a company created to serve the health care needs of a new planned community, Celebration, created by the Walt Disney Company near Orlando, Florida. The town of Celebration had its origins in one of Walt Disney's own visions. Disney hoped to create a model city of the future, with education, health care, community services, and technology to match. After a ten-year study that engaged dozens of futurists, the Disney Company broke ground on the 4,900-acre community in 1994. By the middle of 1996, many people had begun moving into the first of the apartments and 8,000 single-family houses called for in the master plan. (Snyder 1996)

The stated goal of Celebration Health is to create a healthy community model and a healthy company model that can be shared and duplicated while also assisting each person to achieve optimum health.

Owned and operated by Florida Hospital, Celebration Health will stress prevention and a holistic approach to health care, which balances the health of mind, body, spirit, and community. To this end, the main health facility will emphasize lifestyle enhancement above all else. "Whole-person health" is the goal, says Des Cummings, Celebration Health CEO. "We will keep you ambulatory; keep you on your feet. Even if you have a chronic condition, we will help you enjoy a quality of life and a stability of health." (Cummings 1996)

Celebration Health has reserved the Life Enhancement Center's most prominent wing in its initial phase solely for fitness and rehabilitation. That helps Florida Hospital deliver the message that the primary thrust of Celebration Health is prevention—either primary prevention (preventing disease) or secondary prevention (arresting or reversing the progression of disease). "One of our goals," says Cummings, "is to accelerate the adoption in America of a health culture versus an illness culture."(Cummings 1996)

In a wing adjoining the fitness center are the physicians' offices, less prominent, but close enough to the fitness center for physicians to encourage patients into health-maintenance programs available within the facility. The Celebration Health campus will also provide in later phases all necessary inpatient facilities and services for the acutely ill and injured. Patients will begin their relationship with Celebration Health physicians by creating Health MAPS (management action plans) to guide the patient in lifestyle and self-care practices that promote health.

Although Celebration Health's innovations are many, the company's information systems best illustrate the kind of change that many organizations have to look forward to in the coming years. Every home comes outfitted for easy connection to the town's communications system, a fiber-optic network that ties together physicians, hospitals, patients and their families, and pharmacists. Residents can log into the system from home, from the fitness center, and from other locations in town. In essence, Celebration Health, working in partnership with other companies, has created a prototype of the health care world of the future. Residents enjoy a host of leading-edge capabilities, each instantly accessible, that range from health monitoring to health education, wellness and medical care, health decision making, medical literature research, and clinical-practice improvement. (Bezold, Corr, and Morrison 1993)

At home, for example, Celebration patients with chronic health risks or ailments can monitor their own vital signs. Hypertensives can measure their blood pressure; diabetics, their blood sugars. DisneyLink will deliver that data immediately to their physicians' offices. If patients believe their symptoms warrant further attention, they can dial up nurses standing by to answer their questions by phone. If they or the nurses believe they need to see a doctor, they can call their doctors' offices and, with the help of computer-mounted video cameras, obtain a videoconference with a physician online, eliminating a trip to the doctor's office. If a visit is necessary, the patient can call up Celebration's scheduling system to sign up for an office visit.

If residents wish to investigate health concerns on their own, they can tap into literature research or health education software piped to their living rooms over the town's fiber-optic cable. Prostate cancer sufferers might, for example, read articles on medical research or sit back and view full-motion video explanations of risks and outcomes of various treatments. They might click on interviews with fellow cancer patients who can explain their experiences with various kinds of care. They might also tap into online discussions to compare notes in real time with fellow patients. And if they still have trouble choosing the best treatment for themselves, they might call up decision-support software to guide them in their decision making, perhaps with the help of simulations that forecast the range of outcomes for cases similar to theirs.

When Celebration residents become ill and need a doctor or hospital bed right away, they will find the Celebration information system plays an equally important role. Physicians with hand-held computers will be able to call up a lifelong record of patients' care. They then maintain a complete online record of examinations and procedures. An extract of pertinent data automatically enters the outcomes research system. According to Larry Presley, chief information officer of Celebration Health, the organization expects to take advantage of neural network technology to comb the research system for hints as to what drug therapies work best. That information would then be delivered to physicians to encourage better prescribing patterns. (Presley 1996)

By information systems alone, Celebration Health has put itself in a position not only to adapt to future discontinuous change but also to thrive on it. The system will put into the hands of patients far more power and resources to guide their own care. It will let residents take greater responsibility for their care, augmenting and, in some cases, even replacing physicians as providers of routine information. It will create a full-blown capability for virtual care in which barriers of time and place melt away. It will supply the vehicle for offering a huge menu of new products—online information, education, decision-support, and counseling services—that aging baby boomers will increasingly demand in coming years. And it will prepare Celebration Health for the globalization of health care, allowing anyone in the world with a phone line to buy the company's services.

Health care managers positioning their enterprises for future success must deal with both continuous and discontinuous changes. Their first task is to accommodate the rapid evolution of health care from a position where clinical professionals control the medical knowledge and employers and governments pay the bills, to one where customers drive the changes. These managers must prepare for the day when the old assumptions disappear altogether. That, in our view, is the day when the consumer takes the reins, when the consumer's knowledge comes from easy access to the knowledge and information that used to be reserved for experts, and when the consumer's power comes from more complete control of health care's purse strings.

Winning health care leaders, like those in so many industries before them, must create their future by delighting the consumer. They must craft new strategies to create consumer value and build new competencies to deliver that value. Equally important, they must guide their people through organizational transformation with newfound change-management skills. That is how they will meet the challenge of creating value—a challenge that, once overcome, will produce a new future that sets the standards for excellence in management and excellence in helping people live longer, happier, and healthier lives.

# REFERENCES

Bezold, Clement, Christopher T. Corr, and Richard Morrison. 1993. *21st century health systems: principles & visions.* Orlando: Celebration Health and the Inter-national Health Futures Network.

Blenden, Bob. 1995. Interview with Susan Vanderpool and Erik Hansen.

Celebration Company and Florida Hospital. N.d. Celebration health. Prospectus.

Clark, Jim. 1996. Speech delivered at Managed Care Executive Forum, Phoenix, Ariz., April 13.

Compton, Ron. 1996a. Memo to Aetna managers. Unpublished document. Aetna Life and Casualty. April 1.

———1996b. Interview with Ken Jennings. April 18.

Cummings, Des. 1996. Interview with Erik Hansen.

McGuire, David. 1996. Aetna, U.S. Healthcare merger could have major effect on MCOs. *Managed Care*, April 5, 1–2, 6.

Morlet, Andrew N., and Susan M. Oliver. 1995. *Health futures: summary*. Thought Leadership Centre. Andersen Consulting. November.

Oliver, Susan, Andrew Morlet, and Janeer Weerasingam. 1995. *Health futures forum*. Andersen Consulting. November.

Pitta, Julie. 1996. Netscape pioneer to go online with health site . . . *Los Angeles Times*, March 5, D1.

Presley, Larry. 1996. Interview with Erik Hansen. March 7.

Snyder, Jack. 1996. Sometime in June, the first residents of Celebration will settle into their new homes. *Orlando Sentinel*, February 18.

# INDEX

# Knowledge is Power

This maxim best describes why Knowledge Exchange (KEX) is dedicated to helping business professionals achieve excellence through the development of programs and products specifically designed to give them a competitive edge.

KEX's divisions include strategic consulting services; executive education, conferences and seminars; and multimedia, book, and online publishing.

The company's publishing division produces books that demystify the Internet, general business, management, and finance as well as audiobooks, videos, and CD-ROMs. KEX books and audiobooks are distributed throughout North America by Warner Books, Inc.

KEX was founded in 1989 by President and CEO Lorraine Spurge. Formerly a senior vice president at Drexel Burnham Lambert (1983-1989), she raised more than $200 billion for companies including MCI Communications, Turner Broadcasting, Viacom, Barnes & Noble, Mattel, and Tele-Communications, Inc.

KEX Chairman of the Board, Kenin M. Spivak, is also Cofounder, President, and Co–CEO of Archon Communications, Inc. He has served as President of the Island World Group; Executive Vice President and COO of MGM/UA Communications Co.; and Vice President of Merrill Lynch Investment Banking. He is also an attorney and a film producer.

**For more information about the company or its products, write**

**Knowledge Exchange LLC**          TEL: 310.394.5995
**Publicity Department**             FAX: 310.394.7637
**1299 Ocean Ave., Suite 250**      E-MAIL: kex@kex.com
**Santa Monica, CA 90401**          WEB: http://www.kex.com

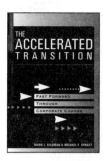

## The Accelerated Transition®

Fast Forward Through
Corporate Change

**MARK L. FELDMAN, Ph.D., and
MICHAEL F. SPRATT, Ph.D.**

An in-depth analysis of companies that have gone
through corporate change, with a concise outline of
proven steps to insure a fast, efficient and successful
transition.

**Hardcover/$22.95** (Can. $28.95)
ISBN 1-888232-28-5

Coming to bookstores in 1997

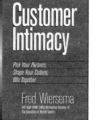

## Customer Intimacy

Pick Your Partners, Shape Your
Culture, Win Together

**FRED WIERSEMA**

Taking business far beyond the concept of good
*customer relations*, bestselling author Fred Wiersema
presents a new way of defining customer relations,
which has produced exceptional sales, profits and
customer satisfaction.

**Hardcover/$22.95** (Can. $27.95)
ISBN 1-888232-00-5
**Audiobook/$14.00** (Can. $17.00)
ISBN 1-888232-01-3
Read by the author

Available in bookstores now

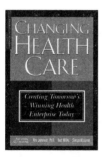

## Changing Health Care

Creating Tomorrow's Winning
Health Enterprise Today

**KEN JENNINGS, Ph.D., KURT MILLER
and SHARYN MATERNA
of ANDERSEN CONSULTING**

An inside look at the health-care industry by a
team from the world's largest consulting firm,
laying out the essential strategies that companies
must follow to survive and thrive in the turbulent
health-care market of tomorrow.

**Hardcover/$24.95** (Can. $29.95)
ISBN 1-888232-18-8

Coming to bookstores in 1997

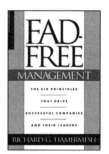

## Fad-Free Management

The Six Principles That Drive
Successful Companies and
Their Leaders

**RICHARD HAMERMESH**

A step-by-step program to implement the six
bedrock management principles that have a
proven track record in helping companies
achieve their goals.

**Hardcover/$24.95** (Can. $29.95)
ISBN 1-888232-20-X

Available in bookstores now

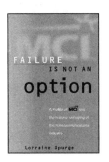

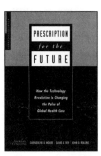

## Failure Is Not An Option

A Profile of MCI

**LORRAINE SPURGE**

A case history that reads like a novel, this is
the story of the tension, suspense, personalities
and brilliant thinking that catapulted MCI from a
start-up to a telecommunications powerhouse,
forever altering the American business landscape.

**Hardcover/$22.95** (Can. $27.95)
ISBN 1-888232-08-0

Coming to bookstores in 1997

## Prescription for the Future

How the Technology Revolution Is Changing
the Pulse of Global Health Care

**GWENDOLYN B. MOORE, DAVID A. REY** and
**JOHN D. ROLLINS** of **ANDERSEN CONSULTING**

In a time of tremendous flux in the health-care industry, this book shows how those who can understand and harness changing technologies will be able
to create the successful health-care organizations of
the future.

**Hardcover/$24.95** (Can. $29.95)
ISBN 1-888232-10-2
**Audiobook/$12.00** (Can. $15.00)
ISBN 1-888232-11-0
Read by the authors

Available in bookstores now

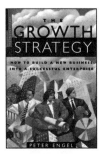

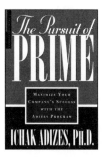

## The Growth Strategy

How to Build a New Business
into a Successful Enterprise

**PETER ENGEL**

A book that entrepreneurs have been waiting for, it
shows businesses how to get beyond the start-up
phase to become professionally managed businesses
that will create true wealth for their owners.

**Hardcover/$22.95** (Can. $28.95)
ISBN 1-888232-30-7

Coming to bookstores in 1997

## The Pursuit of Prime

Maximize Your Company's Success
with the Adizes Program

**ICHAK ADIZES, Ph.D.**

The renowned author shows companies how to
successfully navigate the various growth stages
of a business and reach *prime*—the stage at
which they are most healthy and profitable.

**Hardcover/$24.95** (Can. $29.95)
ISBN 1-888232-22-6

Available in bookstores now

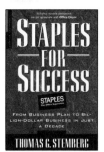

## Staples for Success

From Business Plan to Billion-Dollar
Business in Just a Decade

**THOMAS G. STEMBERG**

Written by the man who made Staples a reality, this
is the gripping story of how a simple idea was
turned into a new, multibillion dollar industry (with
key lessons for those who want to do the same).

**Hardcover/$22.95** (Can. $27.95)
ISBN 1-888232-24-2
**Audiobook/$12.00** (Can. $15.00)
ISBN 1-888232-25-0
Read by actor Campbell Scott

Available in bookstores now

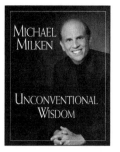

## Unconventional Wisdom

**MICHAEL MILKEN**

The man the *Wall Street Journal* called "the most important financial thinker of the century" shares his
global vision, insight and ideas for the next millennium, providing a guidepost for the next wave of
successful businesses.

**Hardcover/$25.00** (Can. $30.00)
ISBN 1-888232-12-9

Coming to bookstores in 1997

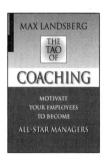

## The Tao of Coaching

Motivate Your Employees
to Become All-Star Managers

**MAX LANDSBERG**

A must-read for anyone who wants to get the
most out of their *human capital*, this book presents
a new way of approaching people management that
will allow your managers to use their time better
while motivating, developing and creating loyalty
among employees.

**Hardcover/$22.95** (Can. $28.95)
ISBN 1-888232-34-X

Coming to bookstores in 1997

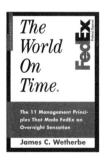

## The World On Time

The 11 Management Principles That
Made FedEx an Overnight Sensation

**JAMES C. WETHERBE**

Learn how Federal Express became a phenomenal
success and discover the eleven innovative management strategies they employed, which have set the
standard for the way businesses manage time and
information, handle logistics and serve customers.

**Hardcover/$22.95** (Can. $27.95)
ISBN 1-888232-06-4
**Audiobook/$12.00** (Can. $15.00)
ISBN 1-888232-07-2
Read by the author

Available in bookstores now

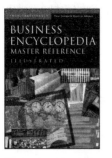

## Business Encyclopedia: Master Reference

**KNOWLEDGE EXCHANGE EDITORIAL BOARD**

The ultimate business tool and the ultimate business gift, this illustrated reference book provides a wealth of information and advice on eight critical disciplines: accounting, economics, finance, marketing, management, operations, strategy and technology.

**Hardcover/$45.00** (Can. $54.00)
ISBN 1-888232-05-6

Available in bookstores now

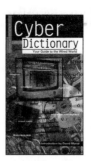

## CyberDictionary

Your Guide to the Wired World

**EDITED AND INTRODUCED BY DAVID MORSE**

In clear, concise language, CyberDictionary makes sense of the wide-open frontier of cyberspace with information useful to the novice and the cyber-pro alike.

**Trade Paperback/$17.95** (Can. $21.95)
ISBN 1-888232-04-8

Available in bookstores now

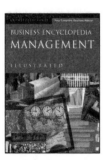

## Business Encyclopedia: Management

**KNOWLEDGE EXCHANGE EDITORIAL BOARD**

Volume two of the Business Encyclopedia series, this book is an essential management tool providing in-depth information on hundreds of key management terms, techniques and practices—and practical advice on how to apply them to your business.

**Hardcover/$28.00** (Can. $34.95)
ISBN 1-888232-32-3

Coming to bookstores in 1997

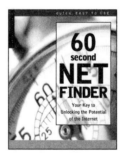

## 60-Second Net Finder

**AFFINITY COMMUNICATIONS AND KNOWLEDGE EXCHANGE EDITORIAL BOARD**

For people who want information from the Internet and want it now, this book shows where to find anything you want, in sixty seconds or less.

**Trade Paperback/$24.95** (Can. $29.95)
ISBN 1-888232-26-9

Coming to bookstores in 1997

# Free Tote with Purchase of Three Books!*

**I'd like to purchase the following books.**

Number of copies

_____ *60-Second Net Finder*

_____ *Business Encyclopedia:*
*Master Reference*

_____ *Customer Intimacy*
_____ *Also available as an audiobook*

_____ *CyberDictionary*

_____ *Fad-Free Management*

_____ *Prescription for the Future*
_____ *Also available as an audiobook*

_____ *Staples for Success*
_____ *Also available as an audiobook*

_____ *The Pursuit of Prime*

_____ *The World On Time*
_____ *Also available as an audiobook*

Name_____E-mail _____

Company_____Title_____

Address_____

City, State, Zip _____

Telephone _____Fax _____

Form of payment:

❏ Check (payable to **Knowledge Exchange, LLC**)          ❏ Credit card

Card # _____Exp. Date _____Card type _____

Cardholder's signature: _____

**Tell us more about yourself:**

| Occupation | Where do you buy business books? | How many business books do you buy a year? | Age Group |
|---|---|---|---|
| ❏ Management | | | ❏ 18–24 |
| ❏ Marketing | ❏ Bookstore | ❏ 0–3 | ❏ 25–34 |
| ❏ Finance | ❏ Mail Order | ❏ 4–10 | ❏ 35–49 |
| ❏ Administrative | ❏ Warehouse Store | ❏ 11–15 | ❏ 50–over |
| ❏ Sales | ❏ Other | ❏ 16 or more | |
| ❏ Other | | | |

**Knowledge Exchange** products are available wherever books are sold.
To order by fax, photocopy this page and fax to 714.261.6137
or call toll-free to order with your credit card.

## Telephone **1.888.394.5996** or Fax **1.714.261.6137**

*Offer expires Dec. 31, 1997 or while supplies last.

Shipping and handling is $4.95 for the first book, $1 for each additional book, $2 additional for each *Business Encyclopedia*. Shipping is via Priority Mail. California residents please add 8.25% sales tax.